101

Sports Nutrition Tips

Susan Kundrat, MS, RD, LD

To allie —
Let nutrition be the
key to "super-fueling" your
body! Good luck!

D1502418

★★★★★
COACHES
≡ CHOICE™

Disclaimer

Every effort was made to provide the most up-to-date material at the time of publishing. However, new and emerging information is coming out continuously. The information contained in this book is provided as general nutrition information and not meant to take the place of professional medical advice. The author and publisher specifically disclaim any liability arising from the use of any information in this book. For specific health concerns or professional advice, a qualified health care professional should be consulted.

ISBN: 978-1-58518-901-4
Library of Congress Control Number: 2004109692

Book layout: Bean Creek Studio
Cover design: Bean Creek Studio

Coaches Choice
P.O. Box 1828
Monterey, CA 93942
www.coacheschoice.com

Dedication

To Vicki — your ideas, dedication,
and constant support have made this book possible.

Acknowledgments

I would like to thank all of the athletes I've been privileged to work with during my career as a sports and wellness nutritionist. Being a part of your success on and off the playing field has been the greatest highlight of my career. Also, my thanks go out to the coaches, athletic trainers, exercise physiologists, and other professionals I've worked closely with, especially Carol Kennedy, MS, and Melinda Flegel, MS, ATC/L, my mentors and colleagues early on in fitness and wellness. I thank my colleagues who provided their insights and encouragement, especially Linda Purcell, Joan Christian, Cathy Leman, RD, and Jenna Bell-Wilson, PhD, RD. In addition, I thank the undergraduate and graduate students in dietetics and kinesiology who have been a part of the background work on this book. Special thanks go to my editors at Healthy Learning. Lastly, thanks to my family for their encouragement, especially to Mom for passing on her love of sports.

Introduction

This book is written for serious athletes, weekend warriors, coaches, athletic trainers, exercise physiologists, personal trainers, parents, teachers, and anyone looking for fast, well-researched nutrition tips for exercise and performance. Most books on sports nutrition are written more academically—they offer great information, but at times they are difficult to sift through for practical tips. *101 Sports Nutrition Tips* provides the most up-to-date information, condensed into an easy reference you can take with you wherever you train or compete.

After 15 years of working with athletes of all ages on nutrition programs to enhance their sports performance, I know athletes are a motivated group. Finding quick ways to improve times, increase strength and endurance, and stay healthy all season long are key goals. In *101 Sports Nutrition Tips*, I've added special features including tables, charts, and bulleted lists that will help you find information easily and put what you learn directly into practice. In addition, my favorite websites are included in Tip #101 so you can continue your quest for information on nutrition and health on the web.

Lastly, when you're fueling your body for performance, you want to be able to visualize and make sense of the amounts of food you are purchasing, preparing, and eating. The idea is to think not in terms of numbers, but of items like golf balls, baseballs, and hockey pucks. And figuring weight measures in milligrams, grams, and ounces is as easy as eating beans and rice.

Sporting Portions	Additional Tips
2 tablespoons of peanut butter = 1 ping pong ball	1 teaspoon = the tip of your thumb
2 ounces of cheese = 1 golf ball	3 teaspoons = 1 tablespoon
1 cup of fruit, veggies, pasta, or rice = 1 baseball	4 tablespoons = 1/4 cup
2 cups of fruit, veggies, pasta, or rice = 1 softball	8 fluid ounces = 1 cup
5 ounces of meat = 1 tennis ball	4 cups = 1 quart = 1 liter
1 bagel = 1 hockey puck	

Making Sense of Milligrams, Grams, and Ounces: Think Beans and Rice
1 milligram = 1/33 of a piece of dry, medium-sized white rice
1 piece of dry, medium-sized white rice = 33 milligrams
1 gram = 30 pieces of dry, medium-sized white rice
1 ounce = 840 pieces of dry, medium-sized white rice
1 dry, medium-sized red kidney bean = 500 milligrams
1 gram = 2 dry, medium-sized red kidney beans
1 ounce = 56 dry medium-sized red kidney beans

Foreword

No topic receives more discussion, or raises more questions, among my athletes than sports nutrition. Athletes at every level have heard about the importance of their dietary food intake. However, most are unaware of the major impact that their nutrition choices have on their daily performance. Additionally, most athletes, coaches, and parents recognize that energy levels and body size can affect performance, yet many seek unhealthy shortcuts rather than safe, long-term changes through their diet. This book is a cover-to-cover promotion of safe, performance-enhancing nutrition tips.

It is my pleasure to present to you *101 Sports Nutrition Tips*. This publication translates textbook sports nutrition research into understandable, consumable information that is easy to implement. No doubt coaches, parents, and athletic trainers will recognize and appreciate how practical these nutrition tips can be for improved performance. *101 Sports Nutrition Tips* breaks through the current myths surrounding carbohydrates, protein, fat, hydration, dietary supplements, and many other subjects. This book will absolutely benefit the healthy athlete in every reader and will be an often-utilized addition to my personal library!

> — Tory R. Lindley MA, ATC/L
> Director of Sports Medicine
> Northwestern University

Contents

1

High-Energy Eating

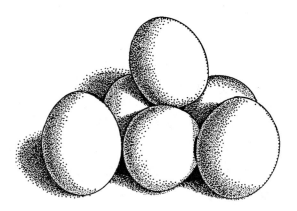

"Think of what you eat as the fuel that gives your body energy to get moving and keep going through your workout, the nutrients to keep your body tuned in high gear, and the fluids you need so your engine runs without overheating."

Tip #1: Assessing Your Sports Nutrition Fitness

Many athletes who are trying to enhance their performance train hard—but often leave out nutrition. They just can't get serious about making the changes in their diet that will give them that extra edge. Are nutrition "roadblocks" keeping you from beating your competition? Take the following quick self-assessment test to find out where you can start making changes. The good news: All of these roadblocks can be overcome by making a commitment to devoting a little time and energy every week to help you meet your goals.

My sports nutrition roadblocks:

____I don't know enough about how the right fuel can improve my performance.

____I'd rather take the "quick fix" than get on a sound nutrition plan for a lifetime.

____I can't seem to eat enough to keep muscle mass on.

____It's too expensive to eat as well as I need to.

____My schedule is so hectic, I don't take time to eat good meals.

____I work out right after work or school, so I don't have a chance to eat a pre-exercise snack to give me energy to work out.

____I don't like water, so I'm often dehydrated.

____I don't have time to get to the grocery store, so I don't have a wide variety of foods available.

____I don't like many different foods, so I end up eating the same foods week after week.

____I don't know how to, or have time to, cook balanced meals.

Tip #2: High-Energy Fuel

You're working out hard, maybe even doing extra workouts or practices to meet your fitness or performance goals. But are you paying close attention to the *fuel* you are putting into your body to improve your performance?

The food you eat is half of the equation when it comes to keeping your body performing at its best. Think of what you eat as the fuel that gives your body energy to get moving and keep going throughout your workout, the nutrients to keep your body tuned to run in high gear, and the fluids you need so your engine runs without overheating. The kind of fuel you fill your tank with will give you the edge when it comes to your sports performance.

For years, researchers in exercise and nutrition have been studying the fuel required for top performance. Whether you're a weekend warrior or train three or more hours a day, you should keep in mind some basics when it comes to high-energy fueling:

- Focus on nutrient-dense carbohydrates as your main energy source. Foods like whole grains, pasta, rice, fruits and juices, beans and peas, vegetables, and milk products are some key sources of carbohydrates for your working muscles. Carbohydrate tips are found in the next chapter.

- Eat the right amount of protein to repair your muscles and tissues. Protein is found in foods like lean meats, fish, eggs, milk and milk products, beans and peas, nuts and seeds, and soy foods. Look for more about this key nutrient in Chapter 3.

- Maintain a reasonable balance of fat in your diet. As you'll see in Chapter 4, fat is an essential part of the sports diet. The key is to get enough fat for energy and health, without overdoing it. Choosing the right kind of fat is also important. Fat is found in foods like nuts, seeds, oils, avocados, margarine, butter, cheese and non-skim milk products, baked goods and desserts, sauces, and salad dressings.

- Keep your body hydrated. Once you get low on fluids, your sports performance can be adversely affected. So, always plan ahead, drink fluids all day long, and have fluids like water and sports drinks available during workouts. For more on fluids, check out Chapter 6.

Tip #3: Energy Balance

Many athletes are missing one very important link when it comes to fueling their active bodies: *energy*. Taking in adequate energy (calories) is of primary importance to you as an athlete. Without enough energy in the system, you'll run out of steam before the end of your workout, or even worse, never be able to gain lean muscle mass. When energy intake isn't adequate, you may burn your own tissue (primarily muscle) for calories, which is exactly what athletes don't want to do!

Sometimes, athletes mistakenly follow a diet that's too low in energy, thinking that it's better to cut calories and lose a few pounds than to overeat. Remember, when you're working out, your body is burning extra calories, and you want to get that energy into your system to fuel your muscles.

Ideally, athletes want to be in *energy balance*, a state where the energy you take in from foods and liquids equals the energy you expend in your day. Energy is burned both in exercise and basic metabolism: the energy to break down food and the energy used in activities of daily living (like taking a shower or walking to the bus stop). Getting

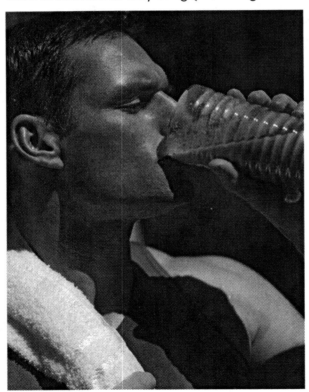

your body in energy balance will help you maintain muscle mass, enhance your immune system, ensure proper growth, and achieve optimum performance.

Tip #4: Calculating Your Energy Needs

The amount of energy (or calories) you need to eat in a day will depend on several factors:

- Body weight
- Fitness level and body composition (i.e., amount of lean body mass)
- Age and gender
- Current sport/fitness routine
- Current eating plan or dietary intake
- Whether you want to maintain, gain, or lose weight

Consult with a sports nutritionist with credentials including R.D. (Registered Dietitian) and education or training in exercise science (see Tip #100) to get an accurate assessment of your energy needs based on your individual needs and goals. To estimate energy needs for *maintaining* your weight, you can use the following calculation based on your current body weight:

Calories Needed Per Day*			
Activity Level	*Calories per pound of body weight (adults)*	*Example: 140 pounds*	*Example: 180 pounds*
Low (infrequent exercise)	13 to 15	1,820–2,100	2,340–2,700
Moderate (30–60 min. 3–4 times/week)	16 to 18	2,240–2,520	2,880–3,240
High (60–90 min. 5+ times/week)	19 to 21	2,660–2,940	3,420–3,780
Very High (90+ min. most days of week)	22 to 25	3,080–3,500	3,960–4,500

Adapted from S. Girard Eberle, 2000, Endurance Sports Nutrition (Champaign, IL: Human Kinetics), p.9.

For *gradual weight loss*, subtract 300–500 calories per day from the total. For *gradual weight gain*, add *at least* 500 calories per day to the total.

*Note: Most athletes need a *minimum* of 1,800–2,000 calories per day, even when decreasing weight. An energy intake that is chronically too low can lead to many unwanted problems, including loss of lean tissue and muscle mass, possible disruption of reproductive function, and increased risk for illness.

Tip #5: Getting the Balance— Top Fuel Sports Pyramid

Finding the right nutrition balance for success can vary from athlete to athlete. The United States Department of Agriculture (USDA) Food Guide Pyramid can serve as a "starting place" for formatting your sports diet. It helps athletes keep balance in mind when choosing an optimum nutrition plan.

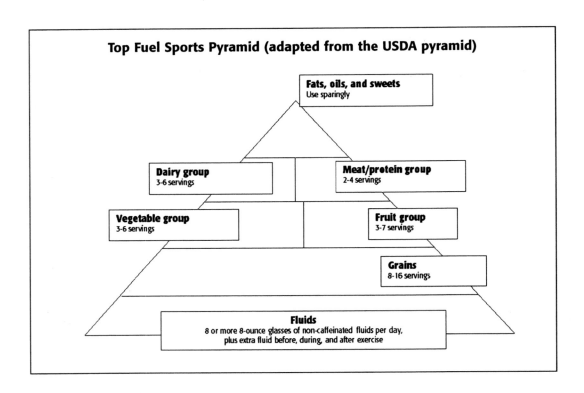

Top Fuel Sports Pyramid (adapted from the USDA pyramid)

Fats, oils, and sweets
Use sparingly

Dairy group
3-6 servings

Meat/protein group
2-4 servings

Vegetable group
3-6 servings

Fruit group
3-7 servings

Grains
8-16 servings

Fluids
8 or more 8-ounce glasses of non-caffeinated fluids per day, plus extra fluid before, during, and after exercise

Tip #6: Recommended Daily Food Servings

What you eat will depend on many factors, including your exercise routine and your food preferences. You can use this simple guide for an estimation of the number of servings from each food group that will meet your recommended needs based on calorie levels. If you eat an average of these recommended servings per day for your calorie level, you'll be on a great start to fueling your body.

Estimated Calorie Needs	Grains	Vegetables	Fruits	Dairy	Meats & Protein	Extras (sweets and fats)
1,800	8	3	3	3	2 (6 oz.)	2
2,200	10	4	4	4	2 (6 oz.)	3
2,600	12	5	5	5	3 (8-9 oz.)	4
3,000	14	6	6	5	3 (10-11 oz)	4
3,400	16	6	7	6	3 (12-13 oz)	5

The higher your energy needs, the more room you have for variety in your training diet. In addition, the harder you train, the more likely you are to benefit from the added energy of sports bars, sports drinks, recovery drinks, and sports gels.

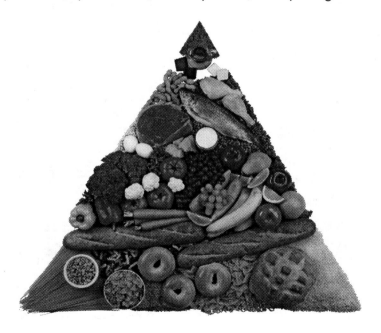

Tip #7: What Counts as a Serving?

Grains (Bread, Cereal, Rice, & Pasta Group)

- 1 slice bread (preferably whole grain)
- 1 tortilla
- 1/2 cup cooked rice, pasta, barley, couscous, or other whole grain
- 1 cup cereal like Wheaties®, Cheerios®, or Bran Flakes®
- 1/2 cup granola
- 1/2 hamburger bun, bagel, or English muffin
- 1 oz. pretzels (1 small bag)
- 1/2 cup potatoes, corn, or peas (starchy veggies)
- 2 small oatmeal cookies
- 1 granola bar or cereal bar

Meat/Protein Group

- 3 oz. cooked lean meat, chicken, turkey, or fish
- 3 oz. lean deli ham, roast beef, or turkey
- 1 oz. meat equals the following:
  - √ 3 oz. tofu
  - √ 1 egg or 2 egg whites
  - √ 1/4 cup egg substitute
  - √ 1/2 cup cooked beans or peas
  - √ 2 tablespoons nut butter (like peanut or soy nut butter)
  - √ 1/4 cup nuts

Vegetable Group

- 1 cup raw, leafy greens (lettuce, spinach, kale, cabbage)
- 1/2 cup chopped raw or cooked vegetables (like broccoli, cauliflower, or green beans)
- 3/4 cup (6 ounces) tomato juice or vegetable juice

Fruit Group

- 1 medium-size apple, orange, or pear (about the size of a tennis ball)
- 1/2 banana or grapefruit
- 2 kiwi fruit
- 1/2 cup chopped, cooked, or canned fruit
- 1/4 cup dried fruit
- 3/4 cup (6 ounces) fruit juice

Dairy (or Dairy Substitutes) Group

- 1 cup milk or fortified soy milk
- 1 cup yogurt or soy yogurt or kefir
- 1 1/2 – 2 ounces cheese or soy cheese
- 1/2 cup cottage cheese or cup ricotta cheese

Extras (Fats and Sweets)

- 1 teaspoon oil, margarine, or butter
- 1 small dessert
- 1 oz. chocolate
- 12 oz. regular soda

Tip #8: Breakfast—The Best Energy Booster

One of the easiest ways to boost your energy level is to start the day with a high-energy breakfast. You don't even have to take much time out of your busy morning. In fact, you don't even have to *sit down* if your time is short (although taking time to sit, relax, and eat is recommended as a way to nourish your body without added stress). The important factor: getting fuel to your muscles, brain, and bloodstream early in the day.

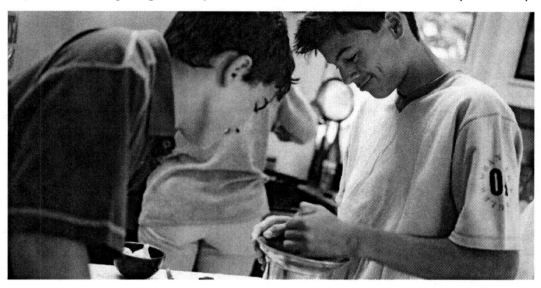

6 Quick Breakfast Ideas

Breakfast #1	*Food group servings*
2 slices whole grain toast with	2 grains
2 tablespoons peanut butter	1 oz. protein
1/2 grapefruit	1 fruit
1/2 cup low-fat cottage cheese	1 dairy
1-2 cups water	extra fluid

Breakfast #2	*Food group servings*
1 cup cooked (1/2 cup dry) oatmeal with 1/4 cup raisins	2 grains 1 fruit
1 cup milk or fortified soy milk	1 dairy
3/4 cup orange juice	1 fruit
1-2 cups water	extra fluid

Breakfast #3	Food group servings
2-egg omelet with 1 cup fresh vegetables	2 oz. protein/2 vegetables
1 whole wheat English muffin	2 grains
with 2 tsp. margarine and jam	2 fats
1 cup melon	2 fruits
1-2 cups water	extra fluid

Breakfast #4	Food group servings
1 bagel with 2 tablespoons low-fat cream cheese	2 grains/1/2 dairy
3/4 cup vegetable juice	1 vegetable
1-2 cups water	extra fluid

Breakfast #5	Food group servings
1 cup vanilla nonfat yogurt	1 milk
1/2 banana	1 fruit
1/2 cup frozen unsweetened strawberries	1 fruit
1 tablespoon protein powder*	1-2 oz. protein
*blend with 3-4 ice cubes for a quick smoothie to go	

Breakfast #6	Food group servings
2 multigrain waffles with	2 grains
2 tablespoons soy nut butter	1 oz. protein
1 banana	2 fruits
3/4 cup grapefruit juice	1 fruit
1-2 cups water	extra fluid

Breakfast Tip: If you're someone who avoids breakfast because you feel hungrier later if you eat it, don't worry. That's normal! When your body gets in "gear," it breaks down nutrients more effectively. All your body is saying is that you are revving up the engine. It's a good sign. Your breakfast may "last" longer if you are sure to include a good protein source (like peanut butter on toast, low-fat cream cheese on a bagel, or yogurt with your cereal). Protein and fat slow down the digestion and absorption of the food you eat at a meal.

Tip #9: Eat Frequently for High Energy

Eating frequently during the day can help you keep your energy up for workouts, work, classes, and all the important things you need to do in your day. To get this benefit, keep your body moving on an "energy surplus" during the day. To do that, always eat when you get up, even if it's something small. In addition, eat frequently throughout the day. In fact, eating frequently enough to register an "energy surplus," where you've eaten more calories than you've burned at various times during the day, may even help keep your body fat percentage down. Some studies suggest eating too few calories can contribute to your body burning fewer calories at rest, higher injury rates, lower bone density, and a higher body fat percentage.

Consider the following example: researchers at Georgia State University evaluated energy balance and body composition in 42 gymnasts and 20 runners, all elite female athletes. The greater the energy deficit (the athletes burned more calories than they were eating throughout the day), the more apt the athletes were to have a higher body fat percentage. The average daily intake of calories was 1,600, and the average predicted energy usage throughout the day was 2,384 calories, so many of the athletes were eating well below their recommended levels. The bottom line: as an athlete, you may perform better and maintain a healthier body composition by eating more often during the day, giving your body needed energy, especially if you've been dieting.

Tips for keeping your energy level high:

- Begin your day with breakfast, even if it's only something small

- Eat a small snack or meal every 3-4 hours during the day

- Don't be afraid to snack after your evening meal. If you're hungry, your body is telling you it needs the energy. Just choose something healthy!

- Listen to your body's hunger cues instead of looking at the clock to determine whether you need to eat.

Tip #10: Three Tips to Help You Eat Often

- Pack a "snack bag" each night to take to work or school. Include foods like trail mix, crackers, fresh fruit, granola bars, energy bars, and juice boxes. If you have the food available, you're much more apt to eat when you're hungry and give your body needed energy.

- Keep a "snack spot" handy in a drawer at work, in your school locker, in your car, or in your backpack. Replenish non-perishable snacks on a weekly basis so you'll always have snack options. Try peanut butter crackers, graham crackers, dried apples or figs, granola bars, and cereal bars.

- Make it a priority to take time for breakfast and lunch. Most people usually eat an evening meal, but these earlier meals often get left behind. Remember, it only takes 5-10 minutes to put together a quick breakfast. At the very least, mix up a powdered instant meal with milk, soy milk, or juice to get you going in the morning. If your time is crunched at lunch, start making a habit of packing a "brown bag" lunch so you don't have to waste time traveling to purchase the meal. Prepare it the night before so it's ready to grab in the morning.

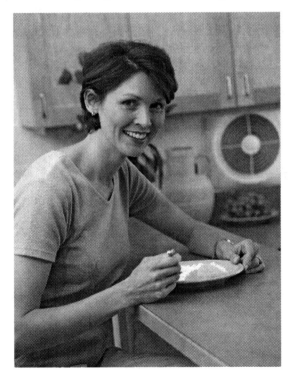

Tip #11: Getting the Right Breakdown of Energy

An athlete's diet is divided into four main categories of energy: carbohydrates, protein, fat, and alcohol. Following is a quick rundown of each energy class and the recommended intake for athletes:

Carbohydrates: Carbohydrates are the starches and sugars found in bread, pasta, cereal, rice, and other grains, fruits and juices, vegetables, milk and milk products, beans, peas, soy foods, and many foods with added sugars like cookies, candies, and soda. Sports drinks and energy bars are often good carbohydrate sources as well. Carbohydrates are the main energy source for your working muscles, and they are also needed to make the brain function. Carbohydrates provide 4 calories per gram to your total calorie intake.

Protein: Protein is found primarily in meats, poultry, fish, milk and milk products, beans, peas, soy foods, nuts, and seeds. Many sports nutrition drinks and bars also contain significant amounts of protein. Grains and vegetables have smaller amounts of protein, but also help the protein add up throughout the day. Protein is crucial for the formation and repair of many of your body's cells, including muscles. Protein also provides 4 calories per gram.

Fats: Fats can be found in many foods, but are abundant in oils, margarine, butter, salad dressings, fatty meats, poultry with the skin, whole milk products, nuts and nut butters, and seeds. Many processed foods such as snack chips, cookies, cakes, candy bars, doughnuts, and muffins can also be high in fat. Fat is essential for helping build body cells, hormones, and other tissues. In contrast to carbohydrates and protein, fat provides 9 calories per gram, over two times the number of calories found in carbohydrates and protein.

Alcohol: Alcohol also provides calories, but limited nutrients. Alcohol is not essential to the body like carbohydrates, protein, and fat, but it is high in calories. Alcohol provides 7 calories per gram, nearly as much as fat.

Your specific nutrient needs will depend on many things, including your body weight, your training schedule, and whether you have other health concerns to take into account. As a general guideline, the recommended breakdown of carbohydrates, protein, and fat for an athlete's diet is:

- 50-70% carbohydrate
- 10-20% protein
- 20-25% fat

To measure the percentages of carbohydrates, protein, fat, and alcohol in a food, use the following equation. The content of each in grams can be found on the food label.

$$\frac{\text{Grams of carbohydrate X 4}}{\text{Total calories}} \quad \text{X 100} \quad = \text{\_\_\_}\% \text{ energy from carbohydrate}$$

$$\frac{\text{Grams of protein X 4}}{\text{Total calories}} \quad \text{X 100} \quad = \text{\_\_\_}\% \text{ energy from protein}$$

$$\frac{\text{Grams of fat X 9}}{\text{Total calories}} \quad \text{X 100} \quad = \text{\_\_\_}\% \text{ energy from fat}$$

$$\frac{\text{Grams of alcohol X 7}}{\text{Total calories}} \quad \text{X 100} \quad = \text{\_\_\_}\% \text{ energy from alcohol}$$

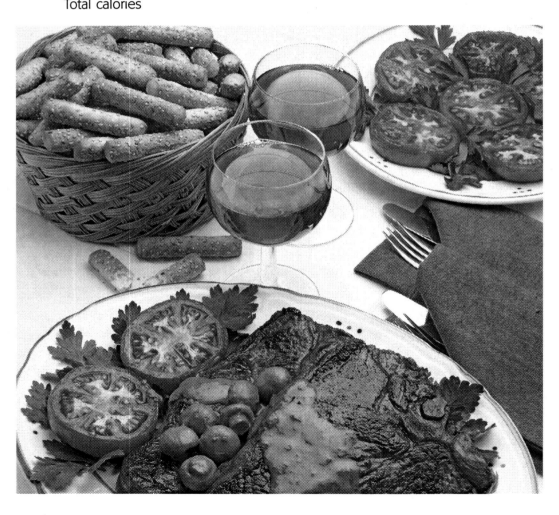

2

Carbohydrates

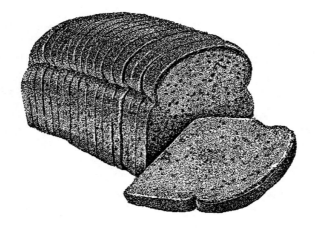

"Carbohydrate is your body's 'energy powerhouse' that fuels your muscles for training and competitions."

Tip #12: Eat a Diet High in Energy-Rich Carbohydrates

Carbohydrate is your body's "energy powerhouse" that fuels your muscles for training and competitions. It is the body's most efficient fuel. You need adequate carbohydrate in your diet to keep your brain and central nervous system running soundly. As an athlete, it's also important to eat a diet high in carbohydrate so your body can limit the use of protein in your body (i.e., your own muscle) as an energy source. Most athletes should aim for a sports nutrition plan with 50-70% of the total calories from carbohydrates. Go for whole grains, fruits, vegetables, and milk products as the main high-energy sources.

More specifically, you can figure your carbohydrate needs based on your body weight and exercise routine. Use the following chart to determine the recommended amount of carbohydrate to eat per day to maximize glycogen (the storage form of carbohydrate) stores and provide your body with adequate energy. The more aerobic your workouts, the greater amount of carbohydrate your body will need.

Recommended Daily Intake of Carbohydrate			
Typical exercise routine	Grams of carbohydrate per pound per day	Example: 140# athlete	Example: 180# athlete
1 hour per day	2.0-3.0	280-420 grams	360-540 grams
1-2 hours per day	3.0-3.5	420-490 grams	540-630 grams
2-3 hours per day	3.5-4.0	490-560 grams	630-720 grams
>3 hours per day	4.0-5.0	560-700 grams	720-900 grams

My weight in pounds = _____ X _____ - _____ grams of carbohydrate per pound per day = _____ - _____ grams of carbohydrate per day.

_____ - _____ grams of carbohydrate per day X 4 calories/gram = _____ - _____ carbohydrate calories per day.

Example: 130-pound athlete exercising 90 minutes per day:

130 lbs. X 3.0 – 3.5 grams per pound = 390-455 grams of carbohydrate per day.

390-455 grams per day X 4 calories per gram = 1,560-1,820 carbohydrate calories per day

Tip #13: Types of Carbohydrates

Carbohydrates can be classified into two types: simple sugars and complex carbohydrates. Carbohydrates from foods naturally high in sugar (fruits) or processed foods (soda, candy, sweets, sugared cereals, table sugar) are generally considered simple sugars. These carbohydrates contain mostly glucose, sucrose, fructose, and high-fructose corn syrup. Fruit is an example of a food high in simple sugars, but also high in nutrients. Complex carbohydrates are made of longer chains of sugars, known as starches and dietary fibers, and are found in whole grains, pasta, beans and peas, vegetables, and some fruits. These foods are generally higher in overall nutrients. The following are carbohydrates you'll find in foods:

Monosaccharides: Glucose, fructose, and galactose are considered the simplest forms of carbohydrate in the diet. Glucose is the main carbohydrate in the blood and forms glycogen, the storage form of carbohydrate. Fructose is found mainly in fruit and honey, while galactose is found in milk.

Disaccharides: Sucrose, lactose, and maltose are made up of two simple sugars. Sucrose is table sugar, while lactose is a sugar found in milk. Many people cannot fully digest lactose and have "lactose intolerance" (see Tip #91). Maltose is made from starch breakdown.

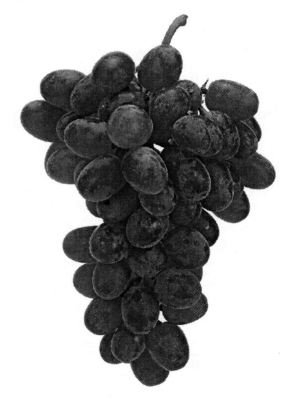

Oligosaccharides: These carbohydrates are short chains of sugars linked together. They include maltodextrin, corn syrup, and high-fructose corn syrup, the main sweetener found in packaged foods.

Polysaccharides: These complex carbohydrates consist of starch and fiber, the non-digestible part of plants.

Tip #14: Top High-Carbohydrate Foods

From the Top Fuel Sports Pyramid (see Tip #5), choose the bottom of the pyramid for the majority of your high-carbohydrate foods. Base your diet on whole grain breads, cereals, pastas, rice, and other grains. Adding fruits, vegetables, skim or low-fat milk products or soy products, and desserts/sweets will provide the bulk of your carbohydrates. Choose natural, high-nutrient carbohydrates whenever possible. Look for "100% whole grain" on the label for the most natural and high-nutrient grains.

Stock your kitchen with these 15 "musts" for carbohydrates:

- 100% whole grain bread
- Brown or whole grain nice
- Potatoes and sweet potatoes
- Dried beans and peas
- Whole grain cereals
- Skim or low-fat milk or soy milk
- Fresh fruits
- Fresh vegetables
- 100% fruit and vegetable juices
- Whole grain pasta
- Yogurt or soy yogurt
- Whole grain pancakes and waffles
- High-energy sports bars
- Sports drinks
- Granola bars and cereal bars

Tip #15: Carbohydrate Amount in Foods

My carbohydrate needs per day: _____ to _____ grams

Food or Beverage	Carbohydrate amount (grams)
1 cup skim milk	12
1 cup Gatorade®	14
1 cup Cheerios®	14
1 cup PowerAde®	19
1 cup All Sport®	20
1 medium apple	20
4 graham cracker squares	22
1 medium banana	25
1 cup orange juice	25
1 cup cooked oatmeal	26
1 cup Sprite®	26
1 cup low-fat chocolate milk	26
2 slices bread	30
1 2-oz. Snickers® candy bar	34
1 cup fruit punch	37
1 toaster pastry	37
12 oz. regular cola	38
1 cup cooked spaghetti	40
1 cup canned corn	40
1 cup cooked white rice	42
4 Fig Newtons®	44
1 cup macaroni and cheese	44
1/2 cup trail mix	45
1 cup raisin bran	47
1 Apricot Clif Bar®	48
1 4-inch cinnamon raisin bagel	49
1 baked potato	50
1 cup fruit yogurt	50
1 cup baked beans	53
1/2 cup raisins	57
5 dried figs	61
1 cup regular granola	64
16 oz. chocolate milkshake	68

Tip #16: Glycemic Index

There has been renewed interest in the glycemic index (GI) of foods in the last several years. The glycemic index is a rating scale that describes how quickly a food is converted to glucose in the blood after it is eaten. The glycemic index is actually a percentage that compares how eating a specific food results in an increase in blood sugar in relation to pure glucose. Glycemic index ranges are from 1-100, with 100 being the rating for pure sugar (glucose).

Eating foods with a lower glycemic index before exercise may moderate the decline in blood sugar (hypoglycemia) that may occur at the beginning of exercise—and therefore possibly reduce the need for carbohydrate as a fuel during exercise, thus increasing available fats for energy. After exercise, carbohydrate may be stored in the muscle better when more high GI foods are consumed. Although keeping an eye on the glycemic index of foods may add some benefit, the most important thing is simply eating or drinking a high-carbohydrate food or fluid in combination with protein as quickly as possible after exercise to replenish muscle carbohydrate, no matter the carbohydrate source (see Tips 66-68).

Many other factors besides the glycemic index of foods can affect how quickly or slowly the carbohydrate is digested and absorbed to be used in the body. Factors such as the total amount of carbohydrate consumed, fiber content, or fat and protein content of the meal or snack will all make a difference. No doubt more research will be done in this area in the years to come.

Tip: Within a balanced diet, choose more of the following lower glycemic index foods (GI<60) *before* exercise:

- Pasta
- Milk
- Yogurt
- Sports bars
- Oatmeal or barley
- 100% bran cereals
- Bananas and grapes
- Apples, pears, and oranges
- Nuts
- Apple juice
- Tomato soup or juice
- Beans and peas (including soybeans)
- Bulgur and barley

Tip: Choose more of the following higher glycemic index foods (GI>60) *after* exercise:

- Baked potatoes and sweet potatoes
- Carrots
- Waffles and bagels
- Sports drinks
- Corn Flakes® Cheerios®, Rice Krispies®
- Graham crackers
- Rice cakes and English muffins
- Honey
- Pineapple and watermelon
- Raisins
- White or wheat bread
- Orange and grapefruit juice
- Pop-Tarts®

Tip #17: Maximizing Glycogen Stores

Glycogen is the storage form of carbohydrates in the body. Glycogen is concentrated in the muscles and the liver. When glycogen is stored, it brings along three-times its weight in water. Glycogen is very important for athletes, as the more glycogen you train your body to store, the higher the amount of this energy-rich source is available before "hitting the wall." Plus, low glycogen stores can result in some not-so-enviable outcomes: fatigue, decreased ability to train intensely, increased risk of injury, and decreased athletic performance. If you train on a daily or almost-daily basis, you will rely greatly on your glycogen stores. Refueling glycogen stores right after workouts is one of the most overlooked—yet beneficial—nutrition keys to enhancing performance.

The total amount of glycogen in the body is only about 1,600 to 2,000 calories, a small amount when you think about it—not nearly as many calories as most athletes burn in a day! For an athlete weighing about 150 pounds, an estimated 400 calories of glycogen are stored in the liver and 1,200 calories of glycogen are stored in the muscle. If you're looking to beat your competition, but find you're out of energy at the end of a race, towards the end of a practice session, or during the last quarter of a game, finding out how to maximize your glycogen stores may be just what you need to get to the next level.

You can maximize the amount of glycogen your body stores by using the following guidelines:

*   Consistently eat enough total calories.

*   Eat a high-carbohydrate diet on a daily basis.

*   Take in plenty of carbohydrates 1-3 hours before workouts and competitions.

*   "Train" your muscles to store glycogen by eating a post-exercise snack high in carbohydrates with added protein after workouts (see Tip #66).

*   Take in carbohydrates (i.e., sports drinks) during workouts.

*   Reduce the rate at which your body uses glycogen by gradually building up your training pace as opposed to going "all out" right away in a workout.

Tip #18: Nutrition During Exercise

During exercise, carbohydrates should be the primary fuel for working muscles. One reason muscles fatigue during prolonged exercise is decreased availability of carbohydrates for energy. During high-intensity, intermittent exercise, such as tennis or soccer, carbohydrates can help keep energy up longer, as well. In one study on tennis players, those provided with a liquid carbohydrate drink (i.e., sports drink) during play improved their ability to hit strokes at the end of prolonged tennis, partly due to the improvement in their running speed. These tennis players also were found to have more explosive strength when they began to get tired than those without carbohydrate. Overall, researchers concluded that carbohydrate intake during prolonged tennis may help players execute technical skills. In soccer players, carbohydrate during exercise has been found to increase running power and the ability to have more contacts with the ball in the second half of the match. These results have been noted in a host of athletes competing in a variety of sports.

During exercise:

- Carbohydrate increases the availability of blood glucose for exercise and helps the body continue to use carbohydrate for energy.

- Carbohydrate also enhances the body's ability to get glucose to the muscles to be used during exercise.

- While training, carbohydrate delays the breakdown of the storage form of glucose (glycogen) in the liver until later in exercise.

- Blood insulin levels rise when carbohydrate is consumed, which helps enhance the muscle's ability to use glucose.

The amount of carbohydrate needed during exercise depends on several factors, including the intensity of exercise and the workout environment. For instance, at low intensities (e.g., moderate cycling), as little as 30 grams of carbohydrate consumed per hour may be adequate, while ingesting 60 grams of carbohydrate per hour may be best with high-intensity exercise (e.g., a basketball game). In cooler weather, less overall fluid (and carbohydrate in a sports drink) may be adequate, while more is needed in hot and humid weather.

Carbohydrate intake should begin early during exercise as opposed to later, when the body is already using up stored glucose. Many an endurance athlete has regretted not drinking a sports drink early enough in the competition. Waiting too long can certainly impact performance negatively.

3

Protein

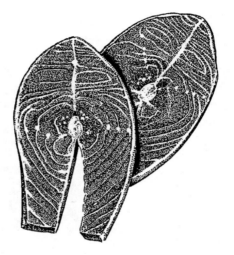

"Without adequate protein, your body can't properly maintain and repair body tissues like muscles, tendons, ligaments, and skin."

Tip #19: Protein Functions

Protein is essential for many functions in your body. In fact, protein can make up nearly half of your body weight. As an athlete, protein helps your body:

*   Provide essential amino acids (protein building blocks) to the cells.

*   Develop new tissues for growth and repair.

*   Make important enzymes, hormones, and antibodies.

*   Keep the cells in fluid balance.

*   Transport substances in the blood.

*   Provide small amounts of energy to the cells.

Without adequate protein, your body can't properly maintain and repair body tissues like muscles, tendons, ligaments, and skin. If your protein intake is low, it may affect how quickly you recover from an injury or illness. In addition, amino acids, the building blocks of protein, contribute as much as 5 to 15 percent of the energy burned during exercise.

Although your muscles do contain protein, simply eating a high-protein diet or taking protein supplements *won't* make your muscles bigger. The winning mix of strength training and eating a diet with *extra* calories (including a variety of foods and a proper mix of protein, carbohydrate, and fat) is the key to successful muscle building.

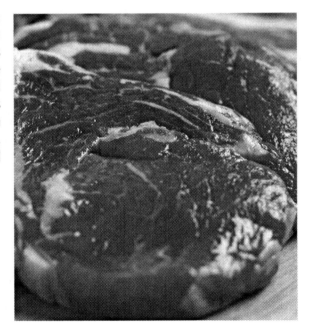

Tip #20: Amino Acids

Amino acids are the building blocks of proteins. Proteins in the diet are made up of 20 different amino acids. Nine of these amino acids are termed "essential" because your body can't make them. You must get them from the foods you eat. To make a complete protein, your body needs all of the nine essential amino acids. Some high-protein foods have all nine of these. These foods are called "complete proteins" and include meat, fish, poultry, milk and milk products, eggs, and soy protein.

Other foods are called "incomplete" proteins because they are missing one or more of the essential amino acids. Combining a variety of "incomplete" protein sources in the diet, as strict vegetarians do, can also provide you with adequate amino acids to build protein. These foods "complement" each other to build proteins. It's generally best to obtain amino acids from foods rather than individual dietary supplements, which may carry risk. For example, if you take too much of one amino acid supplement, you may decrease the body's absorption of other important amino acids. Plus, you may not be getting the protein bonus you're looking for. Many amino acid supplements may have just 10-20% of the total amino acids found in only one ounce of lean meat. Although the amounts of amino acids in supplement vary widely, in one popular amino acid supplement, you would have to take 30 pills to equal the amount of amino acids present in just four ounces of lean roast beef, an excellent food source of protein.

Protein Building Blocks: Amino Acids		
Essential amino acids (must be obtained in the diet)		
Histidine (for infants)	Lysine	Threonine
Isoleucine	Methionine	Tryptophan
Leucine	Phenylalanine	Valine
Non-essential amino acids (the body can make on its own)		
Alanine	Cysteine	Proline
Arginine	Glutamic acid	Serine
Asparagine	Glutamine	Tyrosine
Aspartic acid	Glycine	

Tip #21: Figuring Your Estimated Protein Needs

For athletes, protein needs are based upon your body weight and training routine. Athletes in moderate training may benefit from around 0.5 grams of protein per pound of body weight. For instance, if you run, swim, or bike 3-4 days a week for 30-60 minutes, 0.5 grams of protein per pound of body weight may be appropriate. In heavy training, protein needs may increase to 0.8 grams of protein per pound. In addition, athletes who are working hard to build muscle or are cutting down on calories should take in the upper level (0.8 grams per pound). Intakes above 1.0 gram of protein per pound have not been shown to provide additional benefit for performance. Athletes at risk for not eating enough protein include athletes in a muscle-building stage (i.e., teenage athletes), vegetarian athletes, athletes cutting calories or trying to "make weight," and pregnant athletes.

Protein Needs Based on Body Weight and Exercise Level		
	Maintain muscle mass ➔➔ Gain muscle mass	
	Moderate workouts ➔➔➔➔ Intense workouts	
Weight in pounds	Low end (.5 grams/lb.)	High end (.8 grams/lb.)
100	50 grams	80 grams
120	60 grams	96 grams
140	70 grams	112 grams
160	80 grams	128 grams
180	90 grams	144 grams
200	100 grams	160 grams
220	110 grams	176 grams
240	120 grams	192 grams
260	130 grams	208 grams
280	140 grams	224 grams
300	150 grams	240 grams
	Maintain muscle mass ➔➔ Gain muscle mass	
	Moderate workouts ➔➔➔➔ Intense workouts	

My estimated protein needs per day: _____ - _____ grams

Tip: Eating excess protein well above recommended levels can increase the risk for dehydration. When protein is broken down, its by-products (particularly nitrogen) must be excreted by the body. Water is needed to complete this process. Athletes on a high-protein diet should be sure to drink extra water and keep an eye on urine concentration. Being able to produce normal amounts of clear or light-colored urine is one indicator of a well-hydrated body.

Tip #22: Protein Amount in Foods

Once you've determined your estimated protein needs, you can check out your own diet to find out where you get your protein. Foods high in protein include meats, milk products, foods made with soy protein, selected energy bars and drinks, beans and peas, nuts, nut butters, and seeds. Smaller amounts of protein are also found in grains and vegetables. In fact, most foods (except fruits) from plants and animals contain at least a small amount of protein.

Estimated protein needs per day: _____ - _____ grams

Animal-based Foods	Serving Size	Protein (grams)
Pork and beans	1/2 cup	7
Cheese	1 oz.	7
Milk	1 cup	8
Boiled egg whites	3	10
Fast food small milkshake	1	13
Cottage cheese	1/2 cup	14
Plain yogurt	1 cup	14
Scrambled eggs	3	19
Baked cod	3 oz.	20
Canned salmon	1/2 cup	24
Roast beef or lean meat	3 oz.	24
Pork loin	3 oz.	25
Canned tuna	1/2 cup	26
Chicken breast	3 oz.	26
Turkey breast	3 oz.	26

Tip #23: Vegetarian Protein Sources

If you're vegetarian, or limit your intake of animal foods, you need to be on the lookout for additional protein sources. Even if you don't eat meat, eggs, or milk products, you're not out of luck. Plenty of high-quality foods are available for you to choose from.

Estimated protein needs per day: _____ - _____ grams

Plant-based Food	Serving Size	Protein (grams)
Brown rice	1 cup cooked	5
Whole wheat pita	1 medium	6
Whole wheat bread	2 slices	6
Oatmeal	1 cup cooked	6
Soy milk	1 cup	7
Black beans (cooked)	1/2 cup	7
Soy nut butter	2 tablespoons	7
Sunflower seeds	1/4 cup	7
Spaghetti noodles	1 cup cooked	7
Bagel	1 medium	7
Peanut butter	2 Tbsp.	8
Toasted wheat germ	1/4 cup	8
Green peas	1 cup	8
Peanuts	1/4 cup	9
Tofu	1/2 cup	10
Soy jerky	1 strip serving	10
Veggie burgers	3 oz.	10-20
Soy nuts	1/4 cup	11
Tempeh	1/2 cup	16

Tip: Don't forget to check out canned, frozen, or packaged soups for additional quick protein sources. A couple good options:

Amy's canned Lentil Soup®,
1 cup = 8 grams protein

Nile Spice Black Bean Soup®,
1 package = 12 grams protein

Health Valley Canned Vegetarian Chili®,
1 cup = 14 grams protein

Seapoint Farms frozen Edamame Rice Bowl®,
1 package = 18 grams protein

Tip #24: Portable Protein Sources

Athletes often have a difficult time finding good protein sources when on the road or away from their kitchen. You may think you can only get carbohydrates when on the go, but your working body needs protein, too.

Top 10 Portable Protein Sources

1. Sports bars
2. Trail mix with nuts, seeds, and dried fruit
3. Nuts and seeds (especially soy nuts, almonds, walnuts, pumpkin seeds, and sunflower seeds)
4. Peanut butter, almond butter, or soy nut butter on bread, bagels, or crackers
5. Powdered or canned meal replacement drinks
6. Beef jerky or soy jerky
7. Powdered shake mixes
8. Mozzarella cheese sticks or cheese squares
9. Canned tuna, chicken, or salmon
10. Dehydrated bean soup mixes

High-Energy Snack Mixes

Put together these high-energy snack mixes and store in sealable bags. You'll be able to grab them for a quick snack on your way out the door. Plus, by making your own bags of snack mix, you'll save money in the long run.

Super Trail Mix #1
6 cups Cheerios®, cereal

1 cup soy nuts

1 cup sunflower seeds

1 cup raisins

1 cup dried apples

Makes 16 1/2-cup servings with 180 calories, 20 grams carbohydrate, 8 grams protein, and 8 grams fat per serving.

Super Trail Mix #2
2 cups Cheerios®

2 cups Bran Chex®

2 cups granola

2 cups mini pretzels

1 cup raisins

1 cup salted peanuts

1 cup sunflower seeds

1 cup almonds

1 cup dried apricots

Makes 20 1/2-cup servings with 295 calories, 35 grams carbohydrate, 8 grams protein, and 15 grams fat per serving.

Tip #25: High-Protein Diets

Athletes frequently wonder: "Should I go on a high-protein diet to improve my workouts and increase muscle?" Athletes *do* need more protein than people who are not active or training hard. In fact, athletes may benefit by eating two times the protein that non-athletes need in some cases. For instance, a 160-pound athlete on a dedicated strength training program working to build muscle may require up to 130 grams of protein a day, while a 160-pound sedentary person only needs 60 grams of protein per day. So, athletes' diets should definitely be higher in protein than those of non-athletes.

The problem with some high-protein diets is that they are too low in carbohydrates for working athletes and may be way too high in protein. Some high-protein diets recommend 100 grams of carbohydrate or less per day, nowhere near the recommended amount for working muscles (see Tip #10). And many high-protein diets promote ketosis, a state that occurs in the body when you burn fat in the absence of carbohydrate. Ketosis is not encouraged for athletes looking to find a long-term, balanced nutrition plan.

Another problem: Some high-protein diets are also high in saturated fat, the type of fat that may put athletes at risk for developing heart disease. Diets that are lacking in whole grains, fruits, and vegetables are not complete, as these foods act as "antioxidant powerhouses" in the body (see Tip #33). For maximum benefit from foods for performance, consume at least 8 servings of grains and 6 servings of fruits and vegetables daily for maximum benefit for performance.

High-protein diets may provide inadequate amounts of many vitamins and minerals. These diets may also be too low in fiber, which can lead to constipation and other gastrointestinal problems. In addition, they could potentially increase the risk for gout due to the potential to raise uric acid levels. Lastly, eating a high-protein diet may put you at risk for dehydration, which is already a concern for athletes who are training hard.

As for the beneficial effects of long-term weight loss for people on very high-protein, low-carbohydrate diets, according to the American Heart Association, at present no scientific evidence supports the concepts that high-protein diets result in sustained weight loss, significant changes in metabolism, or improved health. Even if weight is lost in the short term on one of the popular high-protein diets, the question remains whether these diets offer long-term weight loss (for years on end) without additional risk to overall health.

4

Fat

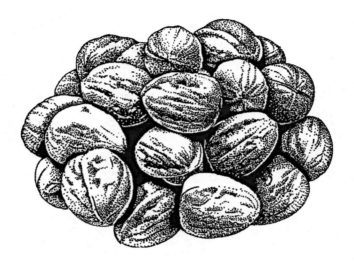

"In addition to providing a concentrated energy source, fat also has important vitamins and essential fatty acids."

Tip #26: Fat Basics

Dietary fat is another key nutrient for the athlete. Although fat often gets a bad rap, it's important to have enough fat (and the right kinds of fat) in your diet for health and performance. During exercise, fat is used as a fuel along with carbohydrate and small amounts of protein. In endurance exercise like long-distance running, swimming, rowing, or biking, fat becomes the primary source of energy for your working body. Many endurance athletes try to train their bodies to utilize more fat and less carbohydrate as energy during exercise to ward off "hitting the wall."

In addition to providing a concentrated energy source, fat also has important vitamins (Vitamins A, D, E, and K, the "fat-soluble vitamins") and essential fatty acids. The fatty acids linoleic acid and alpha-linolenic acid are termed "essential" because the body needs these fatty acids from food for health. The omega-6 fatty acid linoleic acid is found mostly in vegetable oils, including safflower, sunflower, corn, soy, and peanut oil. The omega-3 fatty acid alpha-linolenic acid is provided in seafood, fatty fish like tuna, herring, and salmon, fish oils, canola oil, flaxseed oil, and walnuts.

Fat serves many functions in the body. Fat can be stored for extra energy to be used when the body needs extra fuel. It also makes up cell membranes, keeps certain tissues in your body (including skin) soft and functioning properly, and helps make hormones and nerve cells. In food, fat provides texture and flavor, two important aspects that make eating enjoyable!

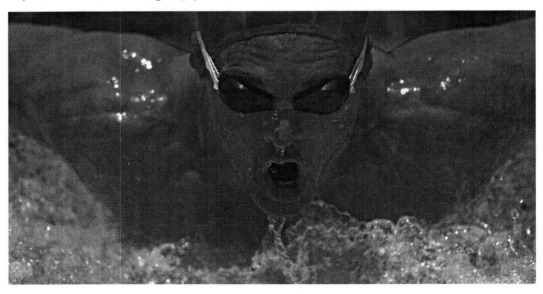

Tip #27: Recommended Fat Intake

Although the "less is better" idea about fat abounds, it's not necessarily true. Taking in about 20 to 25% of your calories from fat is recommended for most athletes. If you're working to gain weight, eating 30% of your calories from fat may help you out. When athletes' energy needs are extremely high (during periods of intense training), even consuming a diet with a fat intake of 50% of total calories in the short-term may not pose problems. In one study, total cholesterol, low-density (LDL) cholesterol, and high-density (HDL) cholesterol were unchanged on a 50% fat diet. But, getting less than 15% of your calories from fat may be linked to a decrease in performance. Ultra-low-fat diets (less than 15% of your calories from fat) have not been found to afford additional benefits to the athlete.

Fat provides more than two times the amount of energy that carbohydrate and protein do (9 calories per gram for fat versus 4 calories per gram for carbohydrate and protein). So, the calories on a high-fat diet can really add up. Some fats are termed "visible fats" because you can see the fat in the foods. For example, salad dressings, oils, butter, and margarine are visible fats. High-fat foods like croissants, doughnuts, cookies, or cheese have "invisible fats," as they are incorporated into foods.

Estimated Fat Needs in Calories and Grams per Day			
Average calorie intake per day	20% of calories from fat	25% of calories from fat	Total grams of fat per day
1,800	360 calories	450 calories	40-50 grams
2,200	440 calories	550 calories	49-61 grams
2,600	520 calories	650 calories	58-72 grams
3,000	600 calories	750 calories	67-83 grams
3,400	680 calories	850 calories	76-94 grams

Tip #28: Fats in Food

Fats in food are generally found as triglycerides, cholesterol, and lipids such as phospholipids and sterols. Triglycerides are three fatty acids attached to a backbone of glycerol. The length of the fatty acids can vary (short, medium, or long-chained fatty acids), as can the amount of saturation. A saturated fatty acid has no double bonds in its structure, while monounsaturated fatty acids have one double bond, and polyunsaturated fatty acids have more than one double bond. It's best to eat a wide variety of foods so you get varied fat sources. Choose more foods low in saturated fat to keep your blood cholesterol levels within a healthy range (Total cholesterol of less than 200 milligrams per deciliter, low-density lipoprotein or LDL at 100 milligrams per deciliter or below). Consume primarily monounsaturated and polyunsaturated fats like canola oil, olive oil, salmon, tuna, sardines, avocados, nuts, and seeds for a heart-healthy diet. Avoid foods high in saturated fatty acids.

Examples of foods high in saturated fatty acids include:

Butter

Whole or 2% milk

Marbled meats, high-fat ground meat, or chicken with the skin

Coconut oil

Palm oil

Shortening

Examples of foods high in monounsaturated fatty acids include:

Canola oil

Olive oil

Sesame oil

Many nuts and seeds

Examples of foods high in polyunsaturated fatty acids include:

Fish oil

Cottonseed oil

Walnuts

Sesame oil

Tip #29: Fat and Immune Status

The immune system is sensitive to fat intake and intense exercise. Athletes sometimes train at very high levels, eat an inadequate diet, and sleep too little. In addition to fat, many essential nutrients that play key roles in immune health have also been found to be low in the diet of some athletes. These nutrients include iron, zinc, and calcium. Thus, some athletes may have suppressed immune systems, which can lead to lower performance levels.

Athletes at highest risk for a lowered immune function are those who train very heavily and chronically undereat or consistently eat too few calories. Many of these athletes eat too little fat along with the lack of calories. Studies have found that limiting fat can negatively affect immune status. In fact, both male and female athletes who exercise at a high intensity for long workouts can safely take in 30% or more of their calories from fat without concerns. For many of these athletes, increasing fat intake can actually enhance performance, as additional calories are able to support training. Moderate-fat diets (i.e., 30% of the calories from fat) are better able to enhance the beneficial effect of endurance training on the immune system than very low-fat diets (<15% of the calories from fat).

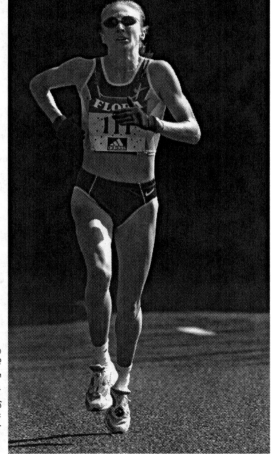

Tip #30: Fat Phobia

Sometimes, athletes become overly worried about gaining body fat, and, in turn, seek to avoid fat in the diet. Aside from putting athletes at a higher risk for a compromised immune system, severely limiting fat intake can be a factor in developing disordered eating patterns. Focusing solely on the fat in a food can be misleading. For instance, if you just look at the fat content of peanut butter, and you are watching every gram of fat, you may mistakenly think it shouldn't be a part of your sports nutrition plan. But, you'll be missing out on important essential fatty acids, iron, protein, zinc, and energy for your workouts. You also might eat many fat-free foods, but find your overall diet lacks nutritional quality.

If you've felt pressure to cut the fat in your diet too low, seek to balance out your nutrition plan gradually. Following are some ways you can slowly reintroduce fat into your plan. You'll have more energy, and your body will get more of a balance of important nutrients. Plus, chances are good that you'll boost your immune system.

- Spread peanut butter or soy nut butter on bread, crackers, or a bagel.
- Top pancakes with sunflower seeds.
- Grate low-fat cheese on your salad.
- Add a slice or two of lean roast beef or ham to your sandwich.
- Bake high-fiber bran muffins with walnuts.
- Mix soy nuts, cereal, and dried apples together for a snack.
- Sprinkle granola over cottage cheese, yogurt, or frozen yogurt.

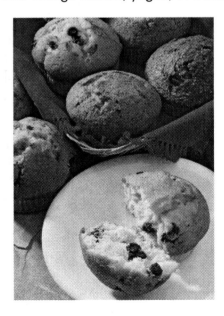

5

Vitamins, Minerals, and Dietary Supplements

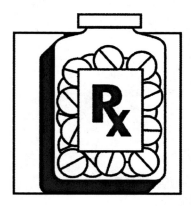

"Completing a sports supplement self-assessment can help athletes determine if a vitamin, mineral, or other supplement is appropriate and will help with training."

Tip #31: Recommended Daily Intakes of Vitamins for Adults

The following table outlines the recommended daily intake for key vitamins for health and performance from The National Academies Food and Nutrition Board. In addition to setting a recommended daily intake level, the board has determined a level which consumers should not exceed. This upper level is not the "ideal" level, but should be considered a level to stay under if you're choosing your diet with one or more vitamins or minerals.

Vitamin	Recommended Daily Intake	Do Not Exceed
Biotin	30 mcg	Not determined
Choline	425 mg for women 550 mg for men	3,500 mg
Folate	400 mcg	1,000 mcg
Niacin	14 mg for women 16 mg for men	35 mg
Pantothenic acid	5 mg	Not determined
Riboflavin (B2)	1.1 mg for women 1.3 mg for men	Not determined
Thiamin (B1)	1.1 mg for women 1.2 mg for men	Not determined
Vitamin A	700 mcg for women 900 mcg for men	3,000 mcg
Vitamin B6	1.3 mg adults 19-50 1.5 mg women over 50 1.7 mg men over 50	100 mg

Vitamin	Recommended Daily Intake	Do Not Exceed
Cobalamin (B12)	2.4 mcg	Not determined
Vitamin C	75 mg for women 90 mg for men 35 mg extra for smokers	2,000 mg
Vitamin D	5 mcg adults 19-50 10 mcg adults 50-70 15 mcg adults over 70	50 mcg
Vitamin E	15 mg (22 IU in natural form; 33 IU in synthetic form)	1,000 mg
Vitamin K	90 mcg for females 120 mcg for males	Not determined

mcg = micrograms; mg = milligrams; IU = International Units

Levels determined by the National Academies Food and Nutrition Board. Log on to www.nap.edu and search for "Food and Nutrition Board" to find the page for specific recommendations for your age and gender.

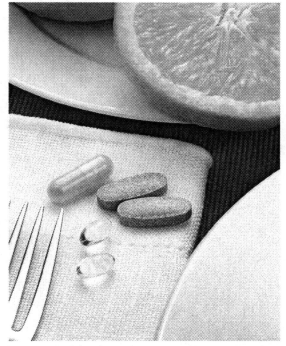

Tip #32: Recommended Daily Intakes of Minerals for Adults

The following table outlines the recommended daily intake and upper limit for key minerals for health and performance from The National Academies Food and Nutrition Board.

Mineral	Recommended Daily Intake	Do Not Exceed
Calcium	1,000 mg adults 19-50 1,200 mg adults over 50	2,500 mg
Chromium	25 mcg for women 19-50 20 mcg for women over 50 35 mcg for men 19-50 30 mcg for men over 50	Not determined
Copper	900 mcg	10,000 mcg (10 mg)
Fluoride	3 mg for women 4 mg for men	10 mg
Iodine	150 mcg	1,100 mcg (1.1 mg)
Iron	18 mg for women 19-50 8 mg for women over 50 8 mg for men Consume twice the recommended amount if vegetarian	45 mg
Magnesium	310 mg for women 19-30 320 mg for women over 30 400 mg for men 19-30 420 mg for men over 30	350 mg*
Manganese	1.8 mg for women 2.3 mg for men	11 mg

*For magnesium the UL is only from supplements; amount naturally found in food and water can be in addition to this number.

Mineral	Recommended Daily Intake	Do Not Exceed
Molybdenum	45 mcg	2,000 mcg (2 mg)
Nickel	Not determined	1.0 mg
Phosphorus	700 mg	4,000 mg adults 19-70 3,000 mg adults over 70
Selenium	55 mcg	400 mcg
Zinc	8 mg for women 11 mg for men Consume twice the recommended amount if a vegetarian	40 mg

mcg = micrograms, mg = milligrams, IU = International Units

Levels determined by the National Academies Food and Nutrition Board. Log on to www.nap.edu and search for "Food and Nutrition Board" to find the page for specific recommendations for your age and gender.

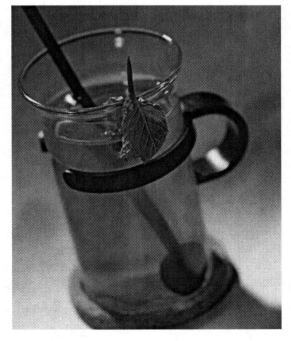

Tip #33: Antioxidants and Exercise

Exercising can be hard on your body's cells, so it's important to eat plenty of antioxidants. These special food compounds can help protect your body's cells from exercise-related damage. Eating foods with plenty of antioxidants may help decrease muscle soreness after hard training sessions or competitions. They may also help keep you healthy all season long, especially when you're training extra hard. Common antioxidants include Vitamins C and E, beta-carotene, and selenium.

To up your antioxidants, eat more of the following antioxidant-rich foods:

- Oranges, tangerines, and grapefruit
- Broccoli, cauliflower, spinach, and asparagus
- Cranberries, strawberries, blueberries, and raspberries
- Purple grapes, green grapes, and raisins
- Pears, peaches, cherries, and apples
- Watermelon and cantaloupe
- Sweet potatoes and yams
- Onions, peppers, and garlic
- Salmon, tuna, and sardines
- Nuts, seeds, and peanut butter

It's actually not that difficult to get in at least six servings of fruits and vegetables a day if you put your mind to it and get in the habit. A quick way to get started on bumping up your servings is to try juicing. It's one fast way to get some concentrated antioxidants in the morning. For example, start off your day with a homemade juice combination like kale, carrot, and orange to give yourself a fast nutrient boost. The following examples show some other ways to plan for at least eight daily servings of fruits and veggies:

Day 1

1. Have a large grapefruit with breakfast (2 servings).
2. Choose a spinach salad with fresh veggies as part of your lunch (2 servings).
3. Add 1 cup of steamed broccoli to your dinner meal (2 servings).
4. Slice an apple and a peach for a snack (2 servings).

Day 2

1. Drink 1 1/2 cups orange juice with breakfast (2 servings).
2. Have a cup of fresh fruit salad with your lunch (2 servings).
3. Choose a veggie stir-fry for lunch (2 servings).
4. For a snack, eat two carrots with hummus dip (2 servings).

Day 3

1. Blend yogurt with 1 cup of frozen berries for breakfast (2 servings).
2. Eat 2 cups of vegetable soup at lunch (2 servings).
3. Eat 1 cup of purple grapes for a snack (2 servings).
4. Have a baked sweet potato with dinner (2 servings).

Including foods high in antioxidants in your sports nutrition plan may pay off in more ways than one. Studies find antioxidants may play an important role in preventing or treating health problems including heart disease, certain cancers (for example, prostate cancer), and cataracts and macular degeneration, two common eye problems. Although more research is on the way, choosing foods high in antioxidants is a good bet.

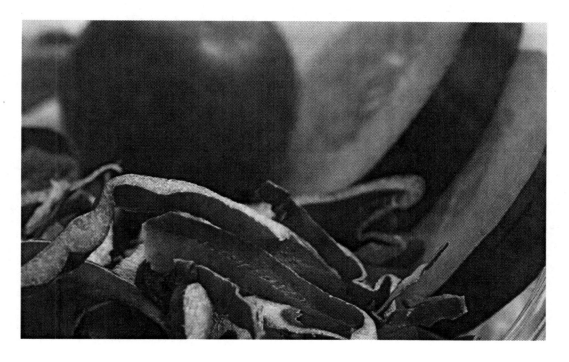

Tip #34: Vitamin C

Vitamin C, also known as ascorbate or ascorbic acid, is an essential water-soluble vitamin and a key nutrient for athletes. It's an antioxidant that may help keep you healthy and decrease your risk of developing certain problems like heart disease and cancer in the future. Vitamin C is also a key nutrient the body uses to form collagen, an essential protein for the development of connective tissue. Vitamin C is important for amino acid metabolism and increases the absorption of dietary iron. Although Vitamin C may not be the "cure-all" it is sometimes touted as, some studies have found it may play an important role in maintaining a sound immune system and may improve symptoms of upper-respiratory infections in some people.

The recommended daily intake for Vitamin C is 75 milligrams for women and 90 milligrams for men. Smokers require an additional 35 milligrams per day. Athletes should consume at least 200-300 milligrams of Vitamin C daily from food to provide an additional amount over the recommended level, but still well below the upper level of 2,000 milligrams per day. Taking in too much Vitamin C in supplement form (over 1,000-2,000 mg per day) may not provide additional benefit, and can also cause nausea, abdominal cramps, and diarrhea. In some susceptible individuals, these high doses could increase the risk for kidney stones.

The best sources of Vitamin C are fruits and vegetables. In fact, eating at least 3 servings from each of these food groups could easily provide 200-300 milligrams of Vitamin C per day, the amount at which the body's blood levels are at least 80% saturated with Vitamin C. Eat foods high in Vitamin C throughout the day so you're giving your working body consistent supplies of this important vitamin all day long.

Recommended intake per day:

75 mg for female athletes   90 mg for male athletes

Additional 35 mg for smokers   Upper level: 2,000 mg per day

Vitamin C in Foods		
At least 100 mg/serving	**At least 50 mg/serving**	**At least 25 mg/serving**
6 medium strawberries	1 kiwi fruit	1/2 grapefruit
1 medium orange	1/4 cantaloupe	1 cup tomato juice
1 cup fresh orange juice	1/2 cup cooked broccoli	1 slice watermelon
1 medium papaya	1/2 cup sweet, green peppers	1 raw avocado
1/2 cup sweet, red peppers	1/2 red or green hot chili pepper	1/2 cup Brussels sprouts
1/2 cup frozen, sweetened peaches	1/2 cup tomato paste	1/2 cup cauliflower
1 cup pineapple juice	1 cup grapefruit juice	1 sweet potato

Tip #35: Calcium

Calcium is one of the most important minerals for an active athlete. It's also the most abundant mineral in your body. Calcium helps build bones and teeth and keeps them strong. Calcium is also crucial for nerve transmission, muscle contraction, and blood clotting. Most athletes need 1,000 to 1,200 milligrams of calcium a day, equal to about 3-4 cups of milk.

Our bodies can build strong bones best before age 18. In fact, it's estimated that 40 to 60 percent of peak bone mass is accrued during the adolescent years. It's important to maximize calcium intake in middle school and high school, the exact time some teens forego high-calcium foods like milk and yogurt. After age 18, you still need ample calcium, as your body is replenishing calcium stores. Calcium is especially key in helping prevent and treat stress fractures.

Your best bets for calcium-rich foods are: milk, yogurt, cheese, pizza, calcium-fortified soy milk and tofu, orange juice with added calcium, broccoli and dark green vegetables, fortified cereals, breads, or cereal bars, and fortified sports bars.

You can check the "Nutrition Facts" food label to find out how different foods stack up when it comes to calcium. You'll find calcium listed as a percentage of the recommended daily amount. Just multiply that percentage by 10 to get the milligrams (mg) of calcium in one serving. For example, if a food has 30% of the recommended daily intake of calcium in one serving, that's 300 milligrams of calcium in one serving (30 X 10 = 300).

Recommended intake per day:

1,000 mg for athletes 19-50   1,200 mg for athletes over 50

Upper level: 2,500 mg per day

Calcium in Foods		
At least 300 mg/serving	**At least 200 mg/serving**	**At least 100 mg/serving**
1 cup yogurt	1 oz. most cheeses	1/2 cup pudding
1 cup skim or 2% milk	1 slice calcium-enriched bread	1 oz. ricotta cheese
1 cup orange or grapefruit juice with calcium (varies)	1 cup 1% or 2% chocolate milk	1 cup ice milk or ice cream
1/2 cup calcium-enriched tofu	1 cup macaroni and cheese	1/2 cup tofu
1 cup cereal with 30% calcium	1 large slice cheese pizza	3 oz. canned salmon w/bones
Sport bars with 30% calcium	1 fortified cereal/granola bar	1/2 cup cooked collards
Soy milk with calcium (varies)	Instant breakfast drinks	1 tablespoon blackstrap molasses

Tip #36: Calcium's Helpers—Magnesium, Phosphorus, and Vitamin D

Calcium certainly doesn't work alone to form strong bones and tissues. The minerals magnesium and phosphorus and Vitamin D are also crucial in the process. Magnesium and phosphorus help build bones, while Vitamin D aids in regulating calcium absorption and deposits into the bone.

Vitamin or Mineral	Recommended intake per day	Food sources
Magnesium	310-320 mg* for female athletes; 400-420 mg for male athletes. Upper limit: 350 mg from supplements and fortified foods	Trail mix, oat bran, bulgur, halibut, spinach, barley, pumpkin seeds, soy foods, nuts, beans, and peas
Phosphorus	700 mg for female and male athletes. Upper limit: 4,000 mg ages 19-70; 3,000 mg over age 70	Meat, fish, poultry, eggs, dairy foods, oat bran, soy foods, wheat flour, many processed foods, soft drinks
Vitamin D	5 mcg*** for ages 19-50; 10 mcg for ages 51-70; 15 mcg over age 70. Upper limit: 50 mcg	Fatty fish like salmon and tuna, fish oils, eggs yolks, butter, Vitamin-D fortified milk and other foods

* milligrams

** International Units

*** micrograms

Tip: To build strong bones, you should ideally eat two times the amount of calcium as phosphorus in a typical day. Sometimes, athletes go overboard on phosphorus and are low on calcium because they forego milk and calcium-fortified drinks for dark soft drinks, which are high in phosphorus.

Tip #37: Iron

Our bodies only hold a very small amount of the mineral iron, but it is an extremely important nutrient for athletes, especially females. Some studies have found that low iron may affect nearly 50% of female athletes in some sports, especially long-distance running. Overall, the prevalence of iron deficiency anemia is thought to be higher in athletic populations (particularly young female athletes), than in non-athletes.

Why is iron so important? Over two-thirds of iron is used in the body to form hemoglobin and myoglobin, compounds that carry oxygen in the blood and muscles. Without adequate iron, cells and muscles don't get the oxygen they need, which can lead to feelings of low energy, and can ultimately impact sports performance. Iron also helps maintain important enzymes to enhance your immune system. It helps produce collagen, important in binding tissues together in your body, and is needed for making other proteins. Vegetarians, children, young women, and adolescents experiencing fast growth are at particular risk for developing low iron stores.

Iron found in meat, poultry, and fish is termed "heme" iron, and is absorbed most easily in the body. Plant-based foods contain "non-heme" iron. A great trick for getting more iron out of your food is to eat a "heme" iron source or a food high in Vitamin C (like fruit or fruit juice) in combination with breads, cereals, pasta, beans, or whole grains to increase the iron absorption. Beware: Coffee, tea, soda, and other caffeinated beverages may decrease the absorption of iron in the diet.

Recommended intake per day:
> 18 mg for women 19-50   8 mg for women over 50 and men
> Upper level: 45 mg

Note: Vegetarians should take in twice the recommended amount for their age group, as non-heme sources are not absorbed as well.

Iron in Foods		
At least 2.0 mg/serving	**At least 1.0 mg/serving**	**Add'l good sources**
3 oz. lean beef*	3 oz. lean ground beef*	Enriched bread and grains
Fortified cereals	3 oz. chicken*	Wheat germ
1 oz. pumpkin seeds	3 oz. lean pork*	Eggs
1/2 cup bran	1 cup cooked enriched pasta	Tofu or fortified soy foods
1 tablespoon blackstrap molasses	1 cup cooked enriched rice	Fish and shellfish*
1/4 cup soy nuts	1/2 cup raisins	Beans and peas
1/2 cup boiled spinach	5 dried prunes	Fig bars
1/2 cup cooked soybeans	1/2 cup canned beans	Nuts and seeds
1/2 cup canned asparagus	1 oz. almonds	Instant breakfast drinks

* heme iron sources

Tip #38: Zinc

Zinc is integral for hundreds of processes and reactions in the body, including wound healing, cell growth and repair, metabolic rate, protein utilization, and enzyme function. It's also an essential nutrient for proper functioning of the immune system. Most of the body's zinc is present in muscle and bone. Nutrition surveys report that many Americans don't consume adequate zinc. Young children ages 1 to 3, adolescents, and the elderly are at greatest risk for low zinc intake. As an athlete, zinc is a very important mineral for your body's proper functioning and resistance to illness. Some of the best sources of zinc are seafood, meats, nuts, eggs, and seeds.

Recommended intake per day:

> 8 mg for women　　　　　11 mg for men
> Upper level: 40 mg

Note: Vegetarians should take in double the recommended amount for their gender, as zinc absorption is lower for those consuming vegetarian diets.

Zinc in Foods	
Food	**Amount of zinc (milligrams)**
3 oz. cooked oysters	74.1
3/4 cup Total® cereal	15.0
3 oz. beef roast	8.7
3 oz. crabmeat	6.5
3 oz. lamb	6.2
1 beef taco	6.1
1 cup trail mix	4.6
3 oz. lean ground beef	4.4
1 roast beef submarine sandwich	4.4
1 cup baked beans	3.8
1/4 cup sunflower seeds	1.8
2 tablespoons wheat germ	1.8
1/4 cup almonds	1.2
2 eggs	1.1
1 cup milk	1.0
2 tablespoons peanut butter	0.9

Tip: Beware of dietary supplements that supply more than the upper limit of zinc set by the Food and Nutrition Board (40 grams/day). The window for optimal zinc intake is narrow and taking in too much has been found to decrease copper absorption.

Tip #39: Vitamin and Mineral Supplements

You may be a candidate for taking extra vitamins and/or minerals to help you achieve your performance goals. So much research comes out nearly every day on different vitamins, minerals, and other nutrients that it's a challenge keeping up with the studies. If you have a particular medical concern, it's important to work with your health care provider or sports nutritionist to learn about new developments that may affect your specific needs.

Of course, food should be the primary source of vitamins and minerals in your diet. Including a variety of foods from all of the food groups will help ensure your body is running strong. But, in many cases, a multivitamin/mineral or specific vitamins and minerals may be helpful. Athletes should take a multivitamin/mineral with 100% of the recommended nutrients for their age and gender to help meet their needs. Think of it as "an extra boost" towards optimum nutrition. You can look at it as a way to bump up your daily nutrients. Check the label for the United States Pharmacopeia (USP) stamp of approval, which guarantees that the supplement contains the declared ingredients in the stated amounts. The supplement should also dissolve properly in your body.

The following list describes some cases when more vitamins or minerals (in addition to a multivitamin/mineral supplement) could be of help:

- If you don't eat animal products, you may need additional iron, zinc, and Vitamin B12.

- If you have food allergies or cannot tolerate certain foods (e.g., milk products), you may be low in the specific nutrients associated with those foods or food groups.

- If you are lactose intolerant, your diet may be low in calcium unless you are choosing other calcium-fortified or high-calcium foods.

- If you are pregnant, you will need to take a pre-natal vitamin that will give you a variety of nutrients including extra folic acid, iron, and calcium.

- If you are a female athlete who experiences heavy menstrual periods or has a history of low iron in your blood, you may need additional iron in a supplement.

Tip #40: Dietary Supplement Self-Assessment

Dietary supplements have been marketed to athletes to do practically everything—increase muscle size and strength, increase endurance, give you more energy, decrease body fat, help you concentrate better, and give you the edge over your opponent. While some supplements may be appropriate, many on the market today are questionable. Currently, the U. S. government does not test dietary supplements for safety and effectiveness, so you must be a "supplement sleuth" yourself or enlist the aid of a sports nutritionist, pharmacist, primary care provider, or other health care provider. Use the following supplement self-assessment to find out if a particular dietary supplement will help you out.

SPORTS SUPPLEMENT SELF-ASSESSMENT

Name of dietary supplement:

Recommended dosage:

Manufacturer:

- Is the supplement legal?
- How does the supplement claim to help me meet my sports goals?
- Can I find solid research to back up these claims?
- Are the recommended amounts of the supplement at appropriate levels?
- What is the safety record for the supplement?
- What are the possible side effects?
- Will the supplement actually help me with the activities and sport(s) I'm participating in?
- Will the company provide me with background information on their testing of supplements?
- Is the cost reasonable within my budget? Does the cost preclude me from buying high-quality foods?
- Does the supplement interfere with any current medications I'm taking?

Tip #41: Searching for Supplement Help on the Web

After completing the self-assessment (Tip #40) on a dietary supplement you're considering, do some background checking with health care providers, via reputable books, or on the web. But, you must be aware that some web sites are simply trying to sell you products, while others provide unbiased, well-researched information. The following sites are highly recommended:

www.naturaldatabase.com — The Natural Medicines Comprehensive Database was released in September 1999. This database is available in either a "free" or "pay" status. It offers an extensive list of herbs, supplements, and, most importantly, brand-name dietary supplements and ergogenic aids. You'll find information about product contents, safety, effectiveness, research, and drug-supplement interactions. This site is highly recommended for its unbiased, researched reviews. Members can access printable patient information sheets on each substance or supplement.

www.mskcc.org/aboutherbs — Sponsored by Memorial Sloan-Kettering Cancer Center, this site's goal is to provide objective information for the public and for health professionals. It offers summaries for each herb, botanical, or supplement, and details about each supplement's makeup, adverse effects, interactions, and potential benefits or problems. The information is provided in an easy-to-navigate format that is also a great tool for athletes and the general public. The short reviews of pertinent research studies on each supplement or herb, an important aspect of choosing a dietary supplement, are especially helpful. The site covers a wide range of supplements.

www.consumerlab.com — This web site provides background information on a variety of dietary supplements. In addition, you'll find reports on many supplements based on purity, truth of labeling, and safety. For a fee, you can also become a member and receive full reports of particular supplements which have met their standards for testing. If you're curious whether a brand-name supplement you are taking has passed the grade, this site is the place to look.

www.supplementwatch.com — This site offers a wealth of background information on a wide range of dietary supplements, including a brief description of the supplement, claims for effectiveness, the theory behind the claims, scientific support, safety information, the value of use, recommended dosage, and references. This site is a quick reference spot for a variety of background information on the supplement you are interested in. You can search supplements by name or by category (e.g., "cardiovascular supplements"). If you pay a yearly fee, you will receive access to additional information.

http://dietary-supplements.info.nih.gov/ — The Office of Dietary Supplements website from the National Institutes of Health offers a wide range of dietary supplement information. You can search the database for recent research studies on a particular dietary supplement or herb, and gather sound, unbiased material to help you make appropriate decisions on dietary supplement use. The main goal of the Office of Dietary Supplements is to support research and disseminate research results in the area of dietary supplements. Updates on supplement safety are also found on this site.

www.herbalgram.org — The website for the American Botanical Council (ABC) provides a wealth of information on herbs. A nonprofit educational and research organization, the ABC offers science-based information to promote the safe and effective use of medicinal plants and phytomedicines. A search engine allows you to find a variety of herb information, including the description of the herb, its chemical makeup, uses for the herb, safety concerns, appropriate dosage, potential interactions with other herbs, and references.

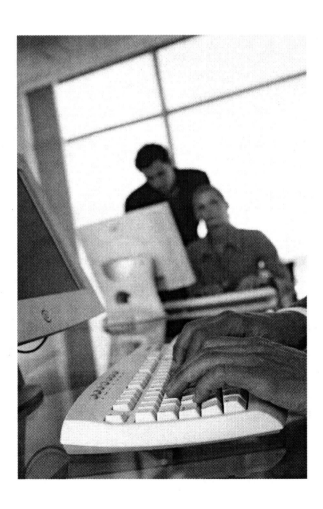

Tip #42: Caffeine

Caffeine has been studied as an ergogenic aid for over 100 years. It is found in the leaves, seeds, and fruits of over 60 different plants. For endurance athletes, caffeine is one of the most widely used stimulants. Caffeine has been found to enhance the ability of endurance athletes to perform, perhaps as a result of caffeine's ability to promote fat metabolism so your body uses less carbohydrate as energy. In some athletes, caffeine may also stimulate the central nervous system to improve performance. Some research has found that limiting caffeine for three to four days before a big race or competition will enhance its effects on the day of the event.

Study results, however, have been mixed. In one study with Belgian tennis players, caffeine was given in addition to carbohydrate to see if it enhanced ability to play tennis, including serving, baseline strokes, and volley performance. Although the carbohydrate was helpful in enhancing play, the caffeine did not provide an additional benefit for stroke quality.

Caffeine is almost completely absorbed once it is ingested. The concentration of caffeine is highest about 45 to 60 minutes after it is taken into the body. As a stimulant, caffeine increases alertness, helps athletes react more quickly, and may help athletes feel they are not having to put out as much effort to see the same benefits compared to exercising without caffeine. However, at high doses, it can work against you, potentially causing fast breathing, high blood pressure, nervousness, an upset stomach and intestinal tract, irritability, and insomnia. Caffeine is also a diuretic, so if you do opt to experiment with it, be sure to stay well-hydrated, drinking extra water and fluids in addition to your typical hydration routine. Like any supplement, be sure your body responds favorably to it in workouts before trying it in a competition. It may be contraindicated in some people with medical concerns like high blood pressure.

Caffeine Content in Selected Foods and Beverages	
Food or Beverage:	**Caffeine amount (milligrams):**
Brewed coffee (1 cup)	65-120 mg
Instant coffee (1 cup)	60-85 mg
Brewed tea (1 cup)	20-110 mg
Most soft drinks with caffeine (12 oz.)	30-60 mg
Dark chocolate (1 oz.)	5-35 mg
Milk chocolate (1 oz.)	1-15 mg

Caffeine is classified as a stimulant by the International Olympic Committee. In large doses (roughly 800 milligrams or more), it is an illegal sports performance supplement. Following are some examples of illegal caffeine doses:

- 7 or more cups of brewed coffee
- 13 or more 12-ounce cans of caffeinated soda
- 4 Vivarin® tablets
- 8 NoDoz® tablets

Tip #43: Chromium

Chromium is considered a trace mineral. We need small amounts of it in our diet to meet the body's needs. The recommended daily intake is 25 micrograms a day for women 19-50 years of age, 20 micrograms for women over 50, 35 micrograms for men 19-50, and 30 micrograms for men over 50. In research studies, dosages used generally range from 200 to 400 micrograms a day. The recommendation for the upper level has not been determined by the Food and Nutrition Board.

Chromium has become a popular dietary supplement for active people and athletes alike. Chromium has been found to affect the action of insulin in the body. For people with diabetes, some studies have found that chromium may help manage blood sugar levels, especially if the body's levels of chromium are low to begin with. Insulin is also important for athletes, as it stimulates the cells to use glucose and amino acids. Although chromium has been touted as a supplement to increase lean muscle mass, several well-designed studies have questioned this thought. Most studies do not support chromium's purported role as a fat burner. Its more relevant role may be aiding in the management of blood glucose levels in people with diabetes because of its effect on insulin. An adverse effect of too much chromium can be chronic renal failure. Most athletes can meet their chromium requirements with a balanced diet that includes some of the following foods high in chromium: eggs, brewer's yeast, baked beans, American cheese, beer, pineapple slices, meat, poultry, fish, mushrooms, and wheat germ.

Recommended intake per day:

25 mcg for women 19-50

20 mcg for women over 50

35 mcg for men 19-50

30 mcg for men over 50

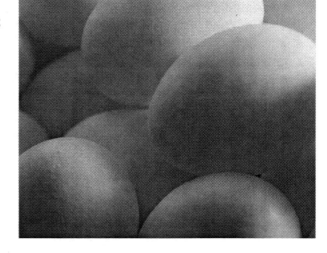

Tip #44: Creatine

Creatine is found in small amounts in foods of animal origin, and may also be made in the liver, pancreas, and kidneys from the amino acids glycine, arginine, and methionine. It is primarily taken as a supplement to increase muscle strength and power in activities such as weight lifting, football, or sprinting. Many (though not all) studies have found creatine may increase muscle power and explosiveness in brief, high-intensity exercise (lasting less than 30 seconds at a time). It may also benefit recovery. However, little evidence supports its use for activities last longer than 90 seconds. Athletes usually take 2-5 grams per day consistently or "load" with 20 grams of creatine daily (four, 5-gram doses) for four to five days and then go back to 2-5 grams per day. If creatine is consumed with glucose (a sugar), it may be slightly more effective. Thus, you may see creatine products combined with carbohydrate.

A common finding in studies involving creatine is an increase in body weight (usually from 2-4 pounds). Although many athletes are looking for weight gain, for some athletes, this weight gain is an unwanted side effect of creatine use, and could potentially slow the athlete down. In well-controlled studies where creatine is taken in appropriate amounts, it appears to be safe. However, many studies have been short in duration (eight weeks or less). Side effects such as diarrhea, muscle cramping, or dehydration have been reported in some athletes. In one study of 52 college athletes, 16 reported diarrhea, 13 had muscle cramps, and seven reported dehydration. If creatine is used, athletes should be careful to stay well-hydrated. Creatine has not been studied in young (ages 18 or younger) athletes; therefore its use in athletes younger than college age is strongly discouraged. Little is known regarding its potential to negatively affect growth and development in young athletes.

Researchers believe vegetarian athletes, who have limited creatine intake from food, may respond most to supplemental creatine. Even for those athletes who consume animal foods, the average intake is about one gram per day, well below the effective doses according to studies. Primary sources in the diet are fish, pork, and beef. A three-ounce portion of beef contains approximately 385 milligrams of creatine, well below the maintenance dose of 2-5 grams (2,000-5,000 milligrams) per day. However, many strength athletes have been successful with maximizing creatine from foods, especially if their calorie needs are 3,000 or more per day. For example, if an athlete eats 8 ounces of lean beef at lunch (two lean hamburgers) and 8 ounces of fish at dinner, that equates to nearly 2 grams of creatine.

Tip #45: Ephedra-free Supplements

With the banning of the controversial supplement ephedra in early 2004 due to concerns about its safety, "ephedra-free" supplements have flooded the market. Many of these supplements are promoted to enhance weight loss, increase energy, speed up metabolism, increase mental alertness, or improve sports performance. Sound too good to be true? Let's take a closer look.

In a recent review of several of the most popular "ephedra-free" supplements on the market. Many of these products contain one or more compounds with caffeine, such as black or green tea, cola nut, guarana, or mate. Several products also contain citrus aurantium (also known as bitter orange or synephrine). Some health professionals have cautioned consumers to be aware that synephrine may have negative effects similar to ephedrine, for example increased heart rate or increased blood pressure. Synephrine is also banned by several sports organizations, including the National Collegiate Athletic Association (NCAA).

Some manufacturers of "ephedra-free" supplements have combined caffeine and synephrine with aspirin-like substances (for example, the herb willow bark) to mimic the "ephedra-caffeine-aspirin stack." Athletes should be aware of these combinations, especially if they are sensitive to caffeine or other stimulants. Plus, several of the supplements reviewed contained large amounts of caffeine, more than the recommended upper level of 300 milligrams per serving.

The bottom line: Although "ephedra-free" products are on the market, some people may react negatively to these supplements. The combination of several "stimulant" or "caffeine-like" compounds in one supplement poses a higher risk than simply drinking a cup of coffee. Most importantly, "ephedra-free" does not necessarily mean "danger-free."

6

Fluids and Hydration

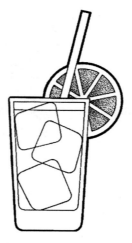

"You want to begin practice or competition in a hydrated state, with your body ready for exercise."

Tip #46: Staying Hydrated

Keeping your body hydrated is one of the most important keys to your success as an athlete. Once you start to become dehydrated, your performance can begin to slip. Dehydration of only two percent of your body weight (i.e., three pounds of sweat lost for a 150-pound athlete) can begin to negatively impact your sports performance. In severe cases of dehydration, heat illnesses can result. In hot conditions, it would not be unusual for an athlete to lose two or three pounds of fluid during each hour of intense exercise. If you only think of drinking water and other fluids *during* exercise, you've started too late. You want to begin practice or competition in a hydrated state, with your body ready for exercise. That way, all you need to do is *replace* lost fluids when you work out, but not make up for a dehydrated body to begin with.

The amount you sweat depends on several factors including the temperature, the humidity, how hard you are exercising, how adapted your body is to exercise, and other individual differences. Some athletes may sweat up to eight cups (four pounds) per hour, while others may sweat very little. On the high end, some collegiate football players have lost 10 pounds in a two-hour practice in the heat and humidity, even when they are trying to drink consistently during the workout! And you don't only lose fluid when you perspire, as sweat also contains sodium, potassium, and small amounts of other minerals like calcium and magnesium.

To stay hydrated, make a habit of keeping water or other non-caffeinated beverages with you all day long. Keep a water bottle or cup of water at your work space, in your backpack, or in your car so you have access to it throughout the day. Shoot for a minimum of 8-10 cups (64-80 ounces) of fluid as your "hydration base" every day. The more you weigh, the greater your fluid needs. By drinking adequate fluids before and during exercise, you'll help your body increase total fluid absorption. Keeping your stomach at an optimal fullness during exercise will help your body empty the fluid better to encourage absorption into your system for use during exercise. Follow these steps:

- Drink at least 2 cups (16 ounces) of fluid when you get up in the morning.
- Drink 2-3 cups (16-24 ounces) of fluid 2-3 hours before exercise.
- Drink 1 cup (8 ounces) of fluid 10-20 minutes before exercise.
- Drink 3/4 cup to 1 1/2 cups (6-12 ounces) of fluid every 15-20 minutes during exercise or during timeouts and game breaks.
- Drink at least an additional 2-3 cups (16-24 ounces) of fluid after exercise or competition to help replace sweat losses.
- Make a point to drink fluids at your next meal to continue to replace those lost in your workouts or competitions.

Tip #47: Monitoring Your Fluid Status

You can do a couple of quick things to keep an eye on your hydration status. Because dehydration can impair your performance quickly and put you at risk for heat illness and injuries, taking a few minutes to self-assess your status is worth the time. Athletes perspire at different rates depending on their biological makeup. Perspiration levels also vary for each athlete depending on the exercise environment. So, try the following two tips to help keep your body running at its best:

- **Monitor your urine output.** If you are hydrated, you should go to the bathroom frequently and have pale or colorless rather than dark-colored urine. If you don't produce much urine, it has a very strong odor, or it's very dark in color, chances are you're dehydrated. Ideally, urine should look more like the color of lemonade, and less like the color of apple juice. Note: Be aware that some medications, foods, vitamins, or dietary supplements may also change the color and odor of your urine.

- **Within two hours of a workout or competition, aim to get back to your pre-exercise weight.** Periodically weigh yourself before and after workouts to ensure you're not losing too much fluid. After exercise, drink at least an additional 2-3 cups (16-24 ounces) of fluid for every pound you've lost in sweat. Remember, losing weight by losing fluid or becoming dehydrated is not the way to get the pounds off. If weight loss is your goal, a sound workout program coupled with a balanced diet is the key. If you're a heavy sweater, make sure to use a beverage containing sodium during workouts (i.e., a sports drink) and eat and drink foods and fluids with sodium after you exercise to replenish the sodium lost in sweat.

To determine how much to drink in fluid ounces to replace fluids lost in sweat, use this simple guide:

How much weight you lost during exercise (1 pound = 16 ounces) plus how much fluid you consumed during exercise (in ounces) equals fluid ounces you need to drink to stay hydrated during exercise.

Example: If you lose 2 pounds in a workout, you lose 32 ounces (2x16). Plus, you drank 16 ounces during the workout. Total fluid needs for the workout = 32 ounces + 16 ounces = 48 ounces, or 6 cups of water or sports drink.

Tip #48: Eat to Hydrate

The most important thing you can do to keep your body well-hydrated is to drink plenty of water and other liquids like sports drinks, juices, and milk all day long and before, during, and after you exercise. Taking in enough fluids is the basis for keeping your body working at its best.

But the foods you eat can also contribute fluid to your sports diet. If you find you have a difficult time meeting your fluid needs, experience frequent muscle cramps, or just don't like water, you're definitely a candidate for adding foods high in fluids to your meals and snacks. Some foods contain 80% or more of their weight in water. So it makes sense to eat more of these foods to stay better hydrated. If you exercise in the heat, live in a hot or dry climate, or just want to keep your body running smoothly, choose more of these foods to aid your performance.

Top 20 Foods That Are at Least 80% Water:

Food	Percentage of water
Cucumbers	96%
Iceberg lettuce	96%
Sweet peppers	92%
Watermelon	91%
Tomatoes	91%
Canned mushrooms	91%
Papayas	89%
Honeydew melon	89%
Onions	89%
Peaches	88%
Pears	88%
Applesauce	88%
Yogurt	88%
Squash	88%
Pasta sauce	87%
Oranges	87%
Cream of Wheat® (cooked)	86%
Canned plums	84%
Mandarin oranges	83%
Cottage cheese	80%

Tip #49: Alcohol

According to the 2000 Dietary Guidelines for Americans, moderate alcohol intake is defined as no more than one drink per day for women and no more than two drinks per day for men, based on the differences between the sexes in both weight and metabolism. A "drink" consists of approximately 15 grams of ethanol, or 12 ounces of regular beer, 5 ounces of wine, or 1.5 ounces of 80-proof distilled spirits.

Contrary to popular belief, drinking beer or other alcoholic beverages is not the best way to rehydrate after hard exercise! Alcoholic beverages contain little carbohydrate, and the alcohol can actually work against you by causing your body to lose fluid and get dehydrated more quickly. So, if you do drink an alcoholic beverage, be sure to accompany it with plenty of water. Drink 8-16 ounces (1-2 cups) of water for every alcoholic drink you consume to help your body stay hydrated.

If maintaining your training weight or losing body fat is your goal, bear in mind that alcohol contains a lot of calories (refer to the chart on the next page). Each gram of alcohol provides 7 calories, nearly twice the number of calories per gram as protein and carbohydrate. Be sure to consider the caloric intake when you are planning your sports nutrition program. When you drink more alcohol, you rob your body of the opportunity to be nourished with more high-nutrient beverages like juices and milk—which, over time, could negatively affect your health and performance.

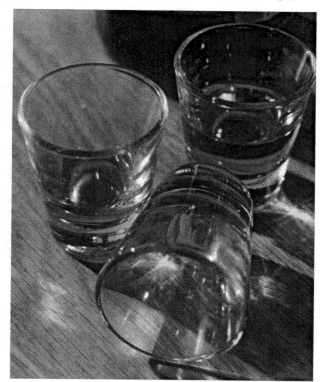

Common Caloric Content of Alcoholic Beverages

Beverage	Amount (ounces)	Calories
Light beer	12	100
Low-carbohydrate beer	12	95
Regular beer	12	140
Beer, stout	12	224
Gin, rum, vodka, or whiskey, 80 proof*	1.5	96
Gin, rum, vodka, or whiskey, 100 proof*	1.5	123
Brandy, cognac	1.5	96
Coffee liqueur, 63 proof	1.5	160
White wine	5	100
Rosé wine	5	105
Red wine	5	106
Wine cooler	12	170
Champagne	5	106
Dessert wine, dry	5	189
Dessert wine, sweet	5	228
Whiskey Sour	4	181
Martini	4	252
Bloody Mary	5	115
Daiquiri	5	240
Margarita	5	330

*80 proof equals 40% alcohol; 90 proof equals 45% alcohol; 100 proof equals 50% alcohol

7

Healthy Weight Gain and Loss

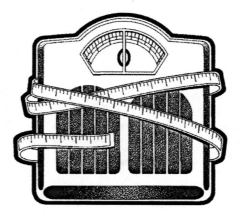

"Set realistic weight loss or weight gain goals of no more than 2 pounds per week for long-term success."

Tip #50: Am I at an Optimum Weight for my Height?

Athletes often wonder if they should gain or lose weight based on the height and weight charts they've seen in their physician's office or posted at the gym. Endurance athletes may find themselves on the lower end of the charts, while those athletes in sports where strength is key may even appear "obese" based on the charts. Using the National Institute of Health's Body Mass Index recommendations (refer to the calculation at the bottom of this page) is a better predictor than the weight charts, but still does not take into account lean muscle mass, bone density, or body fat percentage. Use it as a very general guideline.

The best recommendation is to work with a qualified health professional to assess your body composition, which will give you an estimate of your body-fat percentage in relation to lean body mass. Some of the more commonly employed methods for testing body composition include underwater (or hydrostatic) weighing, bioelectrical impedance analysis, skinfold caliper testing, or air displacement (i.e., Bod Pod®). These measurements are still estimates, although if you are able to have your body composition tested by either underwater weighing or air displacement, the accuracy is better.

How to Figure Your Body Mass Index

$$\frac{\text{Weight (lbs.)} \times 703}{\text{Height (inches)}^2} = \text{Body Mass Index}$$

To check your Body Mass Index online, log on to the National Heart, Lung, and Blood Institute's BMI Calculator at: www.nhlbisupport.com/bmi/bmicalc.htm. According to the National Institutes of Health guidelines:

Underweight = BMI less than 18.5

Normal Weight = BMI 18.5 – 24.9

Overweight = BMI 25.0 – 25.9

Obesity = BMI 30 or greater

Tip #51: Successful Weight Loss Tips

If you're seeking to get in better shape and lose a few pounds in the process, you can do a variety of things to help meet your goals. First off, meet with a sports nutritionist, exercise physiologist, or fitness specialist to correctly determine whether weight loss is appropriate and realistic for you. You can request a body composition measurement to help make this determination. Second, go into the nutrition and exercise plan with a sound goal in mind: long-term weight loss and weight maintenance. By obtaining a sound nutrition program from a qualified and licensed nutrition expert like a registered dietitian, you'll be getting sound advice and recommendations for realistic weight goals.

Quick, short-term weight loss generally isn't successful in the long-term. Even if you lose weight fast, you will probably be losing mostly water (becoming dehydrated) and lean mass, primarily muscle. Plus, if you restrict your diet too much, you'll miss out on important nutrients and energy, risk depressing your immune system, and lack the energy to exercise as well as you'd like. Restrictive dieting can also lead to more severe eating problems like eating disorders.

Tips for Reaching Your Weight-Loss Goals

- Set realistic goals. Don't try to lose too much too fast. Quick weight loss (more than 2 pounds per week for most people) can often result in loss of lean tissue (muscle) or water weight, not fat weight.

- Gradually make changes you can live with. People don't maintain a healthy lifestyle by *dieting*, but by learning how to eat a *healthful diet* week after week and month after month.

- Take your time when eating. The more slowly you eat, the more apt you are to enjoy the food and have it "register" that you actually ate (this process may take at least 20 minutes). People who eat more slowly generally eat fewer calories.

- Plan to eat meals and snacks frequently during the day. Ideally, don't go more than three to four hours without eating. This way, you keep your body well-fueled and prevent those "starvation" feelings that make it difficult to make healthy food choices.

- Get to know your eating style. Do you eat as a result of stressful situations? Do you eat only when you "get a chance" like in the car or while running out the door? Is nutrition a priority in your life? How can you adapt your eating style to allow for a healthful eating plan?

- Monitor what you eat, how you prepare food, what you choose when going out to eat, and when you are hungry. By being aware of what actually goes into your mouth, you can begin to make dietary changes to enhance your lifestyle.

- Keep a food and exercise log. By tracking what you eat, you will help pinpoint where to make changes.

- Keep supportive, healthy people around you! Making lifestyle changes requires a lot of support and encouragement. If you have people in your corner who help you along, that can make all the difference in the world.

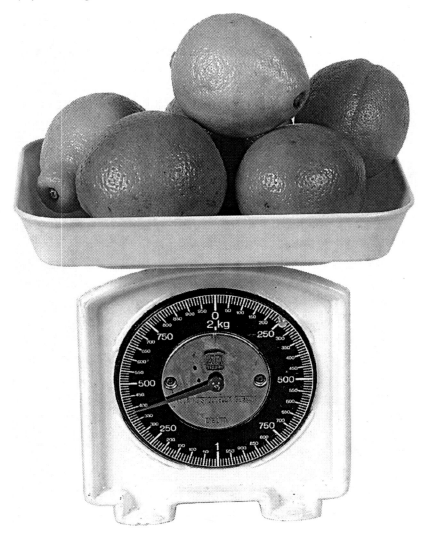

Tip #52: Making Weight for Your Sport

If you're in a sport where you need to make weight to compete at a certain level, you want to make sure you do it in a healthy way. Trying to get down to a weight that's too low for your body may be unrealistic, so be sure your weight goals are reasonable.

For male athletes, a body fat percentage of 5-7% is as low as most athletes should be; for females, 12-15% body fat is generally as low as recommended. It's important to realize that athletes don't always function at their best just because their body fat is low. You may perform better and have more energy at a higher body fat percentage and weight than you initially set as your goal. Many athletes have strived to achieve a lower body fat, only to compromise energy, performance, and health in the process. Depending on the sport and position, many male athletes train best between 10-15% body fat, while females often perform optimally between 15-20% body fat or higher. If you're trying to make weight, consider the following tips:

- Start early. Many successful college wrestlers including some who have become national champions, start tuning their weight in the off-season, not a week or a month before meets. That way, you don't have to cut your calories too much at one time. As a general rule, losing one to two pounds per week is optimal for maintaining muscle mass and strength.

- To lose one to two pounds per week, bump up your exercise enough to burn an additional 2,000-3,000 calories per week while decreasing your food intake by the same amount. For instance, get an additional 20 minutes of exercise a day plus cut out an extra dessert or 20-ounce regular soda during the day.

- Eat small meals or snacks throughout the day, and don't skip meals. This eating plan will keep your energy up for workouts. Shoot for a balanced plate with at least one serving each of a vegetable and a fruit. Include a good protein source like lean meat, fish, or beans and a grain such as pasta, couscous, or whole grain bread.

- Keep your body hydrated all day long. Sometimes we eat because we're actually thirsty, not hungry. Cut down on high-calorie liquids like regular soda, punch, lemonade, juices, juice drinks, and alcohol. Plan for 1-2 glasses of water at each meal.

- Go easy on added fats like salad dressings, mayonnaise, butter, or margarine. French fries or onion rings can also add extra calories.

- Try low-fat snacks like fresh fruit, fresh veggies with nonfat dip, low-fat popcorn, whole grain crackers, low-fat or nonfat yogurt, and frozen fruit bars.

Tip #53: Eating Disorders in Athletes

Most athletes have healthy eating practices. But the pressure of athletics coupled with the array of nutrition misinformation can contribute to the development of eating problems. And although an estimated 90% of people who suffer from eating disorders are female, male athletes can also develop these eating problems. Many different factors could combine to put an athlete at risk for developing disordered eating. Restrictive dieting, long-standing psychological or emotional problems, major life stresses (such as the divorce of parents, moving to a new city, or going through puberty), societal pressures to have a "perfect" body, and individual biochemical factors may all play a role in the development of an eating disorder.

Although not limited to athletes competing in only certain sports, eating disorders tend to be more common in people who play sports that focus on maintaining a smaller or leaner body, mandate a specific weight for performance, or expose the body during competition. Gymnasts, ice skaters, rowers, wrestlers, runners, jockeys, swimmers, divers, cheerleaders, and dancers are examples of some groups of athletes who may be at higher risk because of these factors.

Some athletes may develop a clinical eating disorder such as anorexia nervosa or bulimia nervosa. However, many athletes with eating problems may suffer from some, but not all, of the common symptoms. No matter how "defined" disordered eating is, if it affects your psychological, physical, or emotional health, it's important to seek help from a qualified health professional as early as possible. A combination of psychological counseling, medical attention, and nutritional counseling is important for sound treatment. If you or someone you know is challenged with disordered eating, find a trusted coach, family member, friend, or health professional to confide in and get the support needed to seek help.

Atypical eating habits may be one clue that disordered eating is affecting an athlete. The following questions can help determine if food is part of the problem. The greater number of "yes" answers you have, the more apt you are to benefit from help.

- Do you often eat in secret?
- Do you find yourself constantly counting calories, carbohydrates, or fat grams, to the point where it bothers you?
- Do you avoid eating when you know you are hungry?
- Do you often continue to eat even after you know you are full?
- Do you feel guilty when you eat?
- Are you afraid of gaining weight?
- Do you avoid specific foods or entire food groups?
- Do you think about food, dieting, or weight loss a lot during the day?
- Does your preoccupation with food determine your social schedule?

Tip: For more information about eating disorders and how to find support groups of a health professional specializing in disordered eating, visit the National Association of Anorexia Nervosa and Associated Disorders website at www.anad.org.

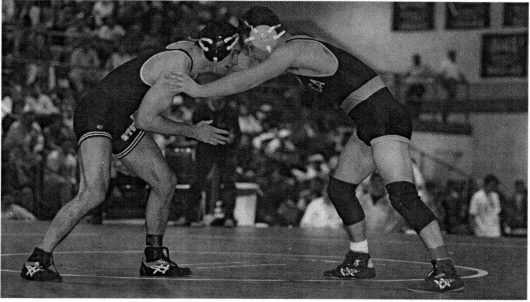

© Todd Rosenberg/Getty Images

Tip #54: The Female Athlete Triad

The female athlete triad is a combination of three interrelated concerns female athletes may develop that can negatively affect health and performance. They are amenorrhea, or loss of a menstrual period for three or more consecutive months; disordered eating; and low bone density, or osteoporosis. When a female athlete suffers from an eating disorder, her dietary intake is often inadequate to meet basic nutritional needs. This low energy and nutrient intake is one reason these athletes may develop bone problems. Low body fat percentage, often associated with amenorrhea, may also be part of the equation. Essential body fat for most women is 12-15% of total weight. But many female athletes may develop loss of menstrual periods above 12-15% body fat. And for some female athletes, this percentage is too low for their bodies to perform at their best.

Several risk factors are associated with the female athlete triad. One or more of these risk factors can make a female athlete more susceptible to developing health problems related to the female athlete triad.

Risk Factors

- Pressure to perform at a very low body weight or body fat composition
- Competition in sports that focus on body size
- Chronic overexercising
- Restrictive dieting or calorie counting
- Being very competitive in a sport
- Unrealistic performance expectations by parents, peers, or athletes themselves to perform well

Warding Off the Female Athlete Triad

You can be proactive in discouraging development of the female athlete triad. Learn how much fuel your body needs for health and competition. Base your fuel intake and training on how your body feels and performs, rather than focusing on body weight or body fat composition. Be aware of the warning signs for developing an eating disorder. If you are a female and your menstrual periods become irregular, get a checkup to find out if the change is due to a medical reason or if it is related to low body fat percentage. If you are a parent or coach, avoid putting too much pressure on athletes or pushing athletes to meet unrealistic or harmful body expectations.

Tip #55: A Plan for Gaining Muscle

To build muscle, you need to combine a sound workout program with at least 3,000 to 4,000 extra calories per week. That's a minimum of 500 extra calories per day on top of what you're already eating at meals and snacks. Many athletes even need 1,000 or more extra calories per day to see results. If you have a naturally high metabolism, it may take even longer to turn food into muscle when balanced with a sound workout plan. Following are some tips to get you going:

- **Maximize "eating opportunities."** Many athletes don't put enough fuel in their bodies because they haven't thought ahead through the day's schedule. By taking easy-to-pack snacks like sports bars, fruit, juices, trail mix, cheese and crackers, and granola bars along during the day, it doesn't matter where you are or what your schedule is—you'll always be able to eat when you get a free minute. Don't be caught hungry and without fuel.

- **Make the most of high-calorie liquids.** Drink a big glass of juice or milk when you get up in the morning. Carry single-serving cans or bottles of high-calorie liquids like grape, cranberry, pineapple, or apple juice with you during the day. This way you can grab a drink when you have a break during the day. Order milkshakes, milk, juices, smoothies, or drinks like lemonade or punch with meals. Blend up a homemade milkshake with ice cream, milk, and frozen fruit before going to bed to boost calories by at least 500 per day.

- **Make time for breakfast.** Just by grabbing a peanut butter sandwich and a banana when you head out the door in the morning, you can add over 400 calories to your daily intake. In one month, that could potentially equal three pounds of weight gain! Since time is often a big issue with athletes on the run, remember that breakfast doesn't need to be eaten sitting down. Before you go to bed, get one step ahead by packing a quick breakfast like a sandwich, a bagel with cream cheese, or sports bar with a 16-ounce fruit juice or milk.

- **Pay special attention to eating a high-energy snack or meal before workouts.** Coming into workouts with fuel in your system helps you work harder and meet your goals faster. Then, plan for a recovery snack after every workout, whether it's lifting, practice, or an aerobic workout. Past-exercise is a crucial time for maximizing muscle recovery (see Tip #66).

- **Don't fall back on weekends.** Sleeping in on the weekends can be a great reward for a long week. But when you're trying to gain muscle mass, you can sleep right through chances to bulk up with solid nutrition. It's not unusual for athletes serious about gaining weight to get up early in the morning to eat breakfast, then head back to bed for a few hours of much-needed sleep, just so they don't miss out on a chance to get in more calories. The bottom like: make a nutrition plan for Saturday and Sunday in addition to weekdays.

Tip #56: High-Calorie Snacks

If you're struggling to put on muscle, keep quick snacks available so you can pump up the calories every day. Try the following energy-packed snacks with over 500 calories each. Start by adding one high-energy snack a day to your normal diet. To increase your calories by 1,000 each day, add two snacks to your routine.

2 cups of a homemade chocolate milkshake

3 cups of crangrape juice drink

4 fig bars and 2 cups of apple juice

1 piece of cheese pizza and 2 cups of grape juice

2 toaster pastries (e.g., Pop Tarts®) and 1 cup of chocolate milk

8 packaged cheese crackers with peanut butter and 2 cups of 2% milk

1 granola bar, 1/4 cup raisins, and 2 cups of pineapple juice

1 cup of fruit yogurt, 4 graham crackers, and 1 banana

1 turkey sandwich and 1 cup of 2% chocolate milk

2 cups of granola cereal and 1 cup of 2% milk

2 packets of instant breakfast drink mixed with 2 cups of 2% milk

A sports bar and 2 cups of chocolate milk or soy milk

A bagel with peanut butter and jelly and a banana

A ham and cheese sandwich and 2 cups of orange juice

Tip #57: High-Energy Shakes

Mixing up fruit smoothies or high-calorie shakes can be an easy way to boost your nutrition plan. Therefore, purchasing a hand-held or tabletop blender is definitely worth the investment. To get fast, high-energy nutrition, try the following shake recipes. Drink them between workouts, after workouts (to aid muscle recovery), when you're in a hurry, or as a snack anytime to help you get stronger. Each shake recipe provides at least 500 calories.

Smooth Chocolate Shake

1 cup regular vanilla yogurt

1 cup 2% milk

1/4 cup dry skim milk powder

3 tablespoons chocolate syrup

Orange-Peach Smoothie

1 cup orange juice

1 cup vanilla ice cream

1/2 cup frozen peaches

Strawberry Smoothie

1 cup 2% milk

1 packet strawberry Carnation Instant Breakfast®

1/2 cup frozen strawberries

1 cup low-fat vanilla yogurt

3 crushed ice cubes

Banana Energy Shake

1 cup 2% milk

1 packet vanilla instant breakfast mix

1 frozen banana

2 tablespoons peanut butter

8

Sports Drinks and Bars

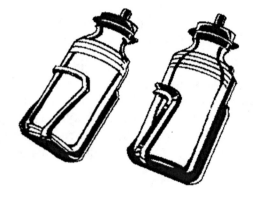

"Consuming sports drinks during exercise can keep athletes hydrated and help them exercise longer, especially in the heat."

Tip #58: Sports Drinks

Consuming sports drinks before, during, or after exercise can help maintain hydration and offer benefits above and beyond water. Because they contain carbohydrates, sports drinks offer your working muscles fast energy to enhance performance. This extra energy in a sports drink has also been documented in many studies to help you exercise longer before you fatigue. In addition, most sports drinks contain sodium and potassium, electrolytes lost in sweat. Adding sodium to sports drinks encourages you to drink more, as it helps drive your thirst. Plus, the addition of electrolytes helps you keep your body's sodium and potassium at optimal levels during training, since you lose these electrolytes when you sweat. Most sports drinks on the market contain around 6-8% carbohydrate, a level that has been found to be absorbed most readily into your bloodstream. A drink that contains too little carbohydrate or too much carbohydrate may not be absorbed and digested optimally.

Studies have found that sports drinks containing sucrose, glucose, or glucose polymers (maltodextrins) have similar effects on exercise performance. However, drinks with only the carbohydrate fructose should be avoided, as fructose is more slowly absorbed from the intestine, and thus gets into the muscles more slowly than other carbohydrate sources. This slow absorption may cause stomach or intestinal upset. Small amounts of fructose as part of the drink's makeup may be tolerated.

The bulk of the research on macronutrients in sports drinks has focused on carbohydrates. Protein, however, has also hit the market in some sports drinks, with claims that it will enhance endurance and aid in muscle recovery. More studies are undoubtedly on the way, but in a recent well-designed study on eight well-trained cyclists completing randomized trials consuming either an 8% carbohydrate, 8% carbohydrate + 2% amino acids, or 10% carbohydrate drink, the addition of amino acids failed to enhance performance of a time trial undertaken at the end of cycling. The most important thing you can do as an athlete is try several brands of sports drinks to see what works best for you. If you like the taste of a sports drink, you'll be more apt to drink more of it in workouts and competition, which can give you the edge over your opponents.

Figuring the Percentage of Carbohydrate in a Sports Drink

On the nutrition label of your favorite sports drink, find the amount (in grams) of carbohydrate per 8-ounce (or 1 cup) serving. Divide the grams of carbohydrate by 240 milliliters and multiply the number by 100 to get the percentage of carbohydrate.

Example: Your sports drink has 14 grams of carbohydrate per 8 fluid ounces (or 1 cup).

14 grams/240 milliliters = .058

.058 X 100 = 5.8% or approximately 6% carbohydrate

Nutritional Breakdown of Several Sports Drinks (per 8 ounces or 1 cup)

	Energy (calories)	Carbohydrate (grams/)	Carbohydrate (percent)	Sodium (mg)
Accelerade	93	17	7%	127
All Sport Body Quencher	60	16	7%	55
Capri Sun Sport	83	23	9%	59
Cytomax	48	10	4%	50
Endura	60	15	6%	92
Gatorade	50	14	6%	110
Gatorade Endurance	60	15	6%	200
GPUSH G2	70	18	7%	190
GU2O	50	13	5%	120
PowerBar Endurance	70	17	7%	160
PowerAde	70	19	8%	55

Tip: For more detailed information on the science of sports drinks, log onto the Gatorade Sports Science Institute website at www.gssiweb.com. You'll find interesting information about the formation of sports drinks, the research behind sports drinks, and tips for improving performance with nutrition.

Tip #59: Fueling Stop-and-Go Sports

Consuming sports drinks in addition to water can help keep you hydrated and give your muscles energy, especially during practices and competitions lasting longer than 60 minutes at a time. But there may be *another* good reason to include them in your performance plan.

Researchers have found that athletes completing a workout similar to what athletes go through in "stop-and-go" sports like soccer, basketball, football, and tennis were able to concentrate better if they drank a sports drink instead of water. In one study, drinks with carbohydrate ingested before and during an ice hockey game reduced muscle glycogen use per unit of distance skated, which is especially beneficial when several games are played in a day or tournament. And in another study, a sports drink consumed prior to the game, midway during each half, and during a 15-minute recovery period improved athletes' performance in the latter section of a soccer-related test compared to those who drank only water. Drinking a beverage with the optimum amount of carbohydrate, like a sports drink, can also keep you more focused on your game by maintaining your alertness.

The bottom line: The quick energy in a sports drink may be fueling your brain as well as your muscles. By drinking fuel with carbohydrate during exercise, you are getting energy to your brain and your working muscles. This energy can potentially help you think more clearly and make better decisions on the court or field, which translates into improved performance.

Tip: Sports drinks are specially formulated to have the appropriate amount and type of carbohydrate and electrolytes to help you perform at your best. They should be your number one choice. But when you're in a pinch, try the following homemade drink for a quick energizer for workouts. Mix together 1 cup of water, 1 cup of orange juice, and a small pinch of salt.

Tip #60: High-Energy Drinks

Some sports recovery drinks, high-energy drinks, or meal replacement drinks are formulated to provide a good mix of macronutrients (carbohydrate, protein, and fat) and additional vitamins and minerals to pack a nutritional punch. These drinks can serve as a fast drink before or after hard workouts or competitions, especially when it's difficult to carry food with you.

Although some athletes also rely on these types of drinks as replacements for actual meals, that's not the best use for them. They should be used in addition to your meals. Build your sports nutrition plan on whole foods and use these drinks as an added benefit, but not a replacement for a balanced meal. Athletes who drink several sports nutrition shakes a day, but skip meals, will miss out on important natural nutrients especially abundant in lean meats, fruits, vegetables, and whole grains. Although many of these drinks are formulated to provide a good balance of nutrients, they can't totally replace real food in the diet.

If you're interested in using a high-energy drink, try several drinks and flavors to find out which ones you like best and work for your specific sports needs. If you plan to use these drinks before or after competitions or events, first experiment with them at a practice or workout so you'll know how your body reacts and you'll feel confident making them part of your game plan. Many drinks on the market today are pre-mixed and ready to consume. You can also purchase several mixes in dry form to combine with water, milk, juice, or soy milk. Most of these drinks taste best when consumed cold. A breakdown of the nutritional content of several high-energy drinks and mixes is listed on the chart on the next page.

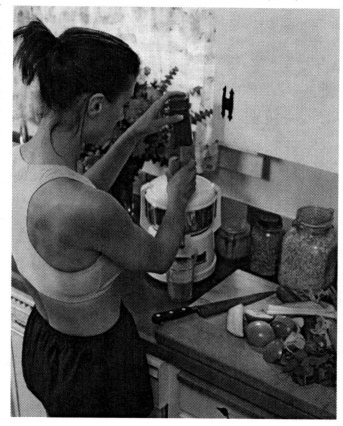

Nutritional Breakdown of Several High-Energy Drinks and Mixes

Product	Amount	Calories	Carbohydrate grams	Protein grams	Fat grams
Boost	8 oz. bottle	240	41	10	4
Boost Breeze	8 oz. can	160	31	8	0
Boost Plus	8 oz. bottle	360	45	14	14
Carnation Instant Breakfast Drink	1 packet	130	27	5	1
Chocolate Milk (1%)	16 oz.	340	56	16	5
Cytomax Pre-Formance	2 scoops	260	35	26	<2
EAS AdvantEdge	11 oz. container	180	28	13	3
EAS Myoplex	1 packet/ 15 oz.	280	24	42	2
Edurox R4	2 scoops/ 12 oz.	270	53	13	1
Ensure Plus	8 oz. can	350	50	13	11
Gatorade Energy Drink	12 oz. bottle	310	78	0	0
Gatorade Nutrition Shake	11 oz. can	370	54	20	8
Genisoy Soy Protein Shake	1 scoop/ 8 oz.	100	0	25	0
GPUSH G4	3 scoops	200	54	<1	0
Hansen's Natural Soy Smoothie	11 oz. container	180	39	7	0
Kashi GoLean	11 oz. container	230	38	15	3
Met-Rx Total Nutrition Drink	1 pkt./ 16 oz.	250	22	37	2
Naturade Total Soy	10 oz.	200	31	13	3
Nesquik Strawberry Milk	16 oz.	400	66	16	0
Power Dream X-Treme Chocolate	11 oz. container	260	48	10	5
Slim•Fast	11 oz. can	220	40	10	3
Snapple-a-Day	11.5 oz.	210	43	7	0
Spirutein Shake	8 oz. container	220	23	22	5
Twinlab Mass Fuel	2 scoops/ 8 oz.	300	58	26	2
Weider Muscle Builder	3 scoops/ 8 oz.	150	21	17	1.5

Tip #61: Energy Bars

You've got a wide variety of energy bars to choose from on the market today, so you should be able to choose a few that you really like to fit into your sports plan. They can provide quick, added energy when you need it most, especially on a training ride, an all-day hike, or between competitions. The carbohydrate helps keep your blood sugar stable and get fuel to your muscles during exercise. Although carbohydrate is generally consumed in liquid form during exercise, solid carbohydrate has been found to produce similar blood glucose and insulin responses. Be sure to experiment with sports bars during workouts or training sessions so you know how your body reacts and you feel comfortable using them. Occasionally, they may cause stomach upset during exercise, especially during high-intensity aerobic workouts or if they are highly supplemented with additional vitamins, minerals, or other nutrients. In addition, they add extra calories to your daily intake, so be sure you're working out hard enough and long enough that you require the extra energy.

Energy bars may contain simple and complex carbohydrates, protein, fat, vitamins, minerals, herbs, antioxidants, and other performance-enhancing components like caffeine or creatine. Many bars are formulated with soy protein and can be a welcome addition to a vegetarian diet. Drink an additional 2 cups (16 ounces) of fluid when you eat an energy bar to help with digestion. Don't rely on them for your primary source of energy, but use them in situations when they may be most helpful to your performance, like an hour or two before a workout, or right after a workout.

Nutritional Breakdown of Several Sports Bars

Product	Size	Energy (calories)	Carbohydrate grams	Protein grams	Fat grams
Balance Bar (chocolate)	1.8 oz.	200	23	15	6
Balance Gold (rocky road)	1.8 oz.	210	26	15	7
Bear Valley Pemmican Bar (carob-cocoa)	3.8 oz.	440	68	16	12
Clif Bar (chocolate chip)	2.4 oz.	250	45	10	5
Clif Luna Bar (nuts over chocolate)	1.7 oz.	180	24	10	4.5
EAS Myoplex Plus Deluxe (chocolate peanut butter)	3.2 oz.	360	44	24	9

Nutritional Breakdown of Several Sports Bars (cont.)

Product	Size	Energy (calories)	Carbohydrate	Protein grams	Fat grams
EAS Myoplex Lite (chocolate fudge)	2.0 oz.	190	27	15	4
Gatorade Energy Bar (peanut butter crunch)	2.3 oz.	250	38	15	5
Genisoy Bar (ultimate chocolate fudge brownie)	2.2 oz.	240	35	14	5
Kashi GoLean Bar (malted chocolate crisp)	2.8 oz.	290	49	13	6
Luna Bar (s'mores)	1.7 oz.	180	26	10	4.5
Met-Rx Bar (fudge brownie)	3.5 oz.	350	52	27	3.5
Met-Rx Protein Plus (chocolate fudge)	3.0 oz.	330	33	32	8
Odwalla Bar (chocolate)	2.2 oz.	240	40	6	6
PowerBar (chocolate)	2.3 oz.	230	45	10	2
PowerBar Harvest (chocolate)	2.3 oz.	260	45	7	5
PowerBar Pria (chocolate honey graham)	1.0 oz.	110	16	5	3
PowerBar Protein Plus (chocolate fudge brownie)	2.8 oz.	270	36	24	5
PR Ironman Bar	2.0 oz.	230	26	16	8
Spiru-tein Bar (peanut butter honey)	1.4 oz.	150	20	10	4
Tiger's Milk Bar (peanut butter honey)	1.2 oz.	150	19	5	6
Verve Meal Bar (chocolate chip peanut crunch)	2.4 oz.	265	41	12	6
Zone Perfect (chocolate caramel cluster)	1.8 oz.	210	20	16	7

9

Nutrition Before and After Exercise

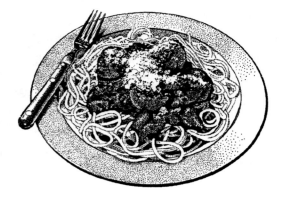

"Timing for pre-exercise and post-exercise fuel is a crucial part of enhancing performance."

Tip #62: Pre-Exercise Nutrition

Nothing is worse than practicing or competing while you're so hungry that your mind is on your stomach instead of your performance. For pre-exercise meals and snacks, a little planning can make a big difference in your athletic success. Choose meals and snacks high in carbohydrates (see Tips #12-18). They'll give you quick energy without slowing you down. Plus, they'll keep your stomach from rumbling. Pre-game meals and snacks are especially important for tournaments or competitions lasting more than an hour. Our bodies handle foods differently. So, test out different pre-game meals before practices or workouts to find out what works best for you.

- Drink plenty of fluids before competition. Dehydration is a simple thing to avoid if you take the time to drink up before and during competition.

- Stick with foods you typically eat before workouts. Avoid trying new foods, eating foods that are too spicy or greasy, or choosing foods that may produce a lot of gas (e.g., beans, broccoli, or high-fiber foods). For most athletes, eating smaller amounts of food before competition works better than eating large quantities. You want to be sure you don't overload your system with too much food.

Timing for pre-game meals and snacks is a key to beating your competition. You'll want to plan the type and amount of food or liquids you take in based on the time you have before you compete. The following chart offers recommendations for what to eat or drink depending on your time schedule.

Time Before Competition	Recommended Food or Liquids	Pre-Game Meal Ideas
30 minutes to 1 hour	Mostly liquids	Sports drink and water
1 to 2 hours	Small snack and liquids	Cereal bar, grapes, apple juice, and water
2 to 3 hours	Small meal and liquids	1/2 turkey sandwich, banana, sports drink, and water
3 to 4 hours	Regular-size meal and liquids	Pasta and meat sauce, salad and low-fat dressing, bread, orange juice, and water

Tip #63: Eating Before Exercise—How the Body Works

Ideally, you'll compete at your best when you have little or no food weighing you down in your stomach. The foods that digest the easiest and fastest are high-carbohydrate foods. Depending on the type and amount of carbohydrate, it may take between one and four hours for these foods to get through the stomach and small intestine.

Sports drinks, which contain simple sugars and are easily digested, get absorbed into your bloodstream and are available as fuel quickly, so you can see why these drinks are great options during exercise. Complex carbohydrates like potatoes, pasta, and bread may take longer to digest (up to three or four hours). You should avoid eating a lot of fat or protein before competition because they both take much longer to digest and move through the small intestine—possibly up to seven hours. In addition, consuming too much fat and protein too soon before competing may contribute to gastrointestinal cramping.

In addition to the *type* of food you eat before competition, the *amount* of food you consume can also significantly affect how your body uses energy. Large meals require many hours to digest and absorb, while smaller meals can get through your system faster. Remember, when the food gets digested and absorbed more quickly, that equates to more energy forwarded to your bloodstream, and eventually to your working muscles—exactly where you want the energy to travel. For pre-game meals, athletes are encouraged to eat a meal that's about two-thirds the size of their normal meals. That way, you aren't going overboard on the amount of food and risking slowing down your performance, especially in the first half or beginning of a competition.

Another way you can help your body do its best to digest and absorb food is to make your pre-game mealtime as relaxed as possible. When you're rushed, nervous, or under stress, your body doesn't utilize food as well as it could, so your body may take a longer time to use the food and get energy to your working muscles. '

Try these tips: Take a few deep breaths before you eat. Give yourself at least 15 minutes to eat your meal. Lastly, plan ahead so you're not in a rush to get to your competition.

Tip #64: Timing of Pre-Exercise Fuel

The timing and size of your pre-competition meals and snacks is not only dependent on the foods and liquids you can tolerate best, but also on your body weight. Studies have found that athletes may perform best when they consume an appropriate amount of energy based on their body size.

For an example, take any athlete who may compete in more than one event, match, or game in a day—a wrestler, a tennis player, a soccer player, or a host of other athletes. Breaks between competitions may be as little as 15 minutes or as long as three or more hours. So, learning what can be consumed to best meet sports goals is essential.

Time before competition	Maximum amount of carbohydrate to take in (per pound)
1 hour	.5 grams
1 1/2 hours	.7 grams
2 hours	.9 grams
2 1/2 hours	1.1 grams
3 hours	1.4 grams

Following is an example of what a wrestler might take in, based on body weight and the time lapse between matches at two different weight classes:

Weight in pounds	Time lapse before match	Sample pre-match fuel
141#	1 hour	Water, 2 cups sports drink, 1 cup cranapple juice
141#	2 hours	Water, 2 cups sports drink, 1 cup cranapple juice, 1 cup grapes, and a sports bar
141#	3 hours	Water, 2 cups sports drink, 2 cups cranapple juice, 1 cup grapes, a sports bar, and a banana
185#	1 hour	Water, 3 cups sports drink, 1 cup cranapple juice
185#	2 hours	Water, 3 cups sports drink, 2 cups cranapple juice, 1 cup grapes, and a bagel with turkey
185#	3 hours	Water, 3 cups sports drink, 3 cups cranapple juice, 1 cup grapes, a bagel with turkey, and an apple

Tip #65: Best Pre-Competition Foods

When choosing pre-competition meals, remember to build your meal or snack around high-carbohydrate foods for the most benefit. Examples of high-carbohydrate foods for pre-competition include bread, cereal, pasta, grains, fruits, juices, vegetables, yogurt, and milk.

Foods to Include in Breakfast

Larger portions of:

Cold cereals
Hot cereals like Cream of Wheat™ or oatmeal
Cereal bars and granola bars
Pancakes and waffles
Toast, English muffins, bagels, and tortillas
Low-fat muffins
Fruit and fruit juice
Nonfat or low-fat milk and yogurt
Nonfat and low-fat soy milk and soy yogurt
Sports drinks
Energy bars and gels
Energy drinks

Smaller portions of:

Poached, boiled, or scrambled eggs
Lean ham, turkey, or chicken
Low-fat sausage or soy sausage
Low-fat bacon, turkey bacon, or soy bacon

Foods to Include in Snacks and Meals

Larger portions of:

Spaghetti and red sauce
Macaroni and cheese
Vegetable soup
Baked potatoes or sweet potatoes
Rice, couscous, quinoa, and other grains
Breads, bagels, pitas, and tortillas
Fruits and fruit juices
Nonfat and low-fat milk and yogurt
Nonfat and low-fat soy milk and soy yogurt
Nonfat and low-fat ice milk and frozen yogurt
Nonfat and low-fat puddings
Low-fat (i.e., mozzarella) cheese sticks
Frozen fruit bars
Sports drinks
Energy bars and gels

Smaller portions of:

Lean meats including turkey, chicken, fish, pork loin, ham, and roast beef
Eggs and soy protein sources (tofu, veggie burgers, soy nuggets)

Tip #66: Post-Exercise Fueling

Scenario: You're working hard to do all the right things with your nutrition plan leading up to a hard practice or competition—eating a solid, balanced diet, taking in a high-carbohydrate meal or snack a few hours beforehand, and drinking plenty of fluids before and during the event. But something crucial is missing. For athletes who are training extra hard, the fuel you take in after exercise can really make a major difference in your performance, too. If you're in the middle of a long season and want to be at your best during the championships, you've got to give your body the nutrients it needs after workouts to gain the edge over your competition. Don't forget to fuel your muscles after exercise!

Post-exercise fuel is especially important if any of the following applies to you:

- Hard daily workouts (1-2 hour practice sessions, long runs, or exhaustive weight training sessions)

- Competition in endurance events (distance races, marathons, bicycling races, or day-long cross-country ski trips)

- Several sports events in one day (an all-day wrestling tourney or several basketball or soccer games in one day)

- More than one workout in a day (two-a-day practices, triathlons, or several daily workouts leading up to a major competition)

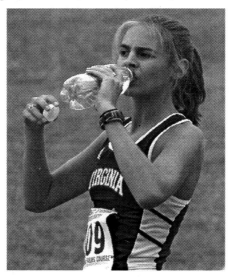

Tip #67: Refueling: Three Lines of Defense

Refueling with Fluids: Your First Line of Defense

The harder and longer you work out, the more fluid you lose through sweat. Studies find that athletes rarely replace all of the fluid lost in sweat by drinking water or a sports drink during exercise. Some athletes don't even replace 50% of the fluids they need. And it's not unusual to lose four or more cups of fluid per hour in sweat when training hard. The more hot and humid the weather, the more likely you are to get dehydrated.

Replacing fluids is the first line of defense for refueling your body after workouts. Drink 2-3 cups (16-24 ounces) of fluid for every pound you lose during practice or competition to help get your body back in balance. Besides water, sweat contains the electrolytes sodium and potassium plus small amounts of calcium, magnesium, and chloride. Most athletes can replenish electrolytes by eating regular meals, as sodium and potassium are usually plentiful in the diet. If you're a heavy sweater or are prone to muscle cramps, be sure to add salt to your food after hard workouts.

Carbohydrates: The Next Step

During exercise, you're relying mainly on stored carbohydrate fuel in the muscle, liver, and blood to energize working muscles. Refueling your muscles right after workouts can help keep your muscles ready to go for the next exercise session, whether later that day or the next day. Refueling right after exercise can also decrease your chance of getting an injury. Think of your muscles as sponges, ready to soak up and store needed nutrients for the next workout.

The Final Step: Adding Protein to the Equation

To re-energize your muscles after a hard workout, you'll also want to focus on protein in addition to carbohydrate and fluids. As a general rule, try to eat or drink a healthy snack within 15-30 minutes of your workout and again in two hours. Even though carbohydrate is the key to supplying your muscles with energy for the next workout, some studies have also found adding protein helps the body store even more energy and recover better than consuming carbohydrate alone.

Tip #68: Refueling Ideas

Several studies have demonstrated that consuming 0.7 grams to 1.5 grams of carbohydrate per kilogram of body weight (approximately 0.3 to 0.7 grams per pound) within the first 15-30 minutes after a workout and again within two hours is beneficial for glycogen recovery. The following examples show how much carbohydrate that equates to based on body weight.

- If you weigh 140 pounds, take in at least 42 grams of carbohydrate after workouts.

- If you weigh 180 pounds, take in at least 54 grams of carbohydrate after workouts.

- If you weigh 220 pounds, take in at least 66 grams of carbohydrate after workouts.

As a general rule, eat at least 50 grams of carbohydrate along with fluids for your post-workout nutrition plan. Most athletes need 50-150 grams of carbohydrate after hard workouts for refueling, depending on body weight. Once you've mastered the high-energy carbohydrates, try adding at least 10-15 grams of protein to the mix. If it's hard for you to eat solid food right after a hard workout, start with something easy like apple, cranberry, or grape juices to get your carbohydrates. Some energy drinks and sports bars also provide a good mix of carbohydrate and protein and are easy to carry with you.

Recovery fuel with at least 50 grams of carbohydrate:

- 1 1/2 cups (12 ounces) crangrape juice
- 2 cups apple or grape juice
- 2 1/2 cups All Sport®
- 4 cups Gatorade®
- 1 cup cranapple juice and 1 granola bar
- 1 cup grape juice, 1 orange, and 3 graham crackers
- 1 cup orange juice and 1 banana

Recovery fuel with at least 50 grams of carbohydrate and 10 grams of protein:

- 1 cup orange juice and 1 cup low-fat fruit yogurt
- 1 cup Gatorade® and 1 PowerBar®
- 1 cup apple juice and 1 peanut butter sandwich
- 1 small fast food milkshake
- 2 cups corn flakes and 1 cup low-fat milk
- 1 1/2 cups soy milk and 1 banana
- 1 Luna Bar® and 2 cups Gatorade®
- 2 cups cranapple juice and 1/2 cup cottage cheese
- 8 oz. Spiru-tein® shake and a bagel

10

Nutrition on the Move

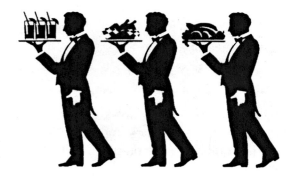

"With a little planning, athletes can eat to fuel performance anywhere—on the road, at tournaments, or even at fast food restaurants."

Tip #69: Dining Out

When eating out at restaurants, choose ones that you know well and that have choices you can trust to complement your training. That way, you can be confident they serve a wide variety of foods so you can make healthy choices. Use restaurant meals as an easy way to get variety in your sports diet by choosing a lean protein source (such as a grilled chicken breast, salmon, lean roast beef, or black beans), a good carbohydrate source (like a baked potato, corn, pasta, or rice), and a salad or steamed vegetables. Following are some additional tips:

- Choose baked, broiled, or steamed meats and main dishes.
- Choose a high-energy grain like pasta, baked white or sweet potatoes, whole grain rice, or couscous.
- Ask for whole grain bread or rolls on the side.
- Go easy on added butter or margarine, oils, salad dressings, or sour cream.
- Choose red sauces for pasta instead of white sauces.
- If you're watching your total calorie intake, choose plain items so you can determine how much extra sauce, dressing, or cheese to add. Many restaurants offer larger-than-life portions, so be prepared to box up part of your meal for the next day's lunch.
- Make a point to order a drink with added nutrients. Go for grapefruit or orange juice, low-fat or nonfat milk or soy milk, or green tea. Always ask for a large glass of water to help you stay hydrated.

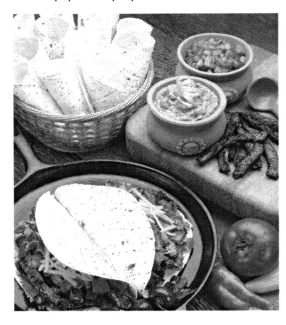

Tip #70: Ethnic Dining Tips

If you're eating in an ethnic restaurant, you can still make healthy nutrition choices. In fact, some ethnic restaurants offer a variety of dishes packed with whole grains and vegetables. Following are healthy choices for three types of ethnic restaurants.

Chinese

- Chicken and vegetables with steamed rice
- Beef and broccoli with steamed rice
- Vegetable lo mein
- Shrimp and vegetables with steamed rice
- Steamed vegetable dumplings

Mexican

- Chicken or beef fajitas with rice, bean, and salsa
- Soft tacos with chicken, beans, or shredded beef
- Bean burritos with vegetables
- Mexican chicken salad with salsa
- Black beans and rice

Italian

- Pasta with marinara sauce, salad, and bread
- Baked chicken breast with pasta and marinara sauce
- Vegetable lasagna, salad, and bread
- Spaghetti, meatballs, and marinara sauce
- Vegetable and Canadian bacon pizza with thick crust

Tip #71: Fast Food Best Bets

When eating out at fast food restaurants, choose foods that will fuel your body with high-energy carbohydrates and protein, but are not too high in total fat. Don't be surprised to find out you can make some healthy choices at fast food restaurants. Look for as many foods from the different food groups as you can to get a balanced meal or snack.

Better Fast Food Choices	
Choose these more often	**Choose these less often**
Bagel with jelly	Biscuits and danishes
Hot cakes (easy on the butter)	Egg sandwiches
English muffins or low-fat muffins	Croissants
Scrambled eggs and lean ham on English muffins	Sausage or bacon on English muffins
Grilled chicken sandwiches	Fried chicken sandwiches
Plain hamburgers or cheeseburgers	Double burgers
Roast beef sandwiches	Fried fish sandwiches
Vegetable pizza	Sausage or pepperoni pizza
Pizza with regular cheese	Pizza with extra cheese
Clear, broth-based soups	Cream soups
Salads with lite dressings on the side	Salads with regular dressings
Chunky chicken salads	Salad bar salads with creamy dressings
Turkey, lean ham, chicken, or roast beef subs	Subs with bologna, pepperoni, or mayo-type salads
Chicken fajitas	Chicken nuggets
Bean burritos	Chimichangas
Mashed potatoes	French fries
Baked potato with chili, salsa, or veggies	Baked potato with butter and sour cream
Grilled or steamed veggies	Fried veggies
Fruit salads and fresh fruit	Fruit pies
Low-fat frozen yogurt or ice milk	Cookies
Juice or low-fat milk	Regular pop
Ketchup, BBQ sauce, pickles, and mustard	Mayonnaise and salad dressing

Tip #72: Healthier Choices at Specific Fast Food Restaurants

Fast food doesn't have to be unhealthy food. Fast food restaurants now have a wide range of fresh salads, lean sandwiches, and other fresh items available. Even if you choose a healthy option, ask for the mayonnaise, sauce, or salad dressing on the side and use it sparingly. Try a few of the following recommended choices:

Arby's
Junior roast beef

Light roast chicken, beef, or turkey deluxe

Roast chicken or grilled chicken salad

Grilled chicken deluxe

Grilled chicken Caesar salad

Asian sesame salad

Burger King
Ham, egg, and cheese bagel

Hamburger or cheeseburger

Whopper junior or chicken Whopper junior

BK veggie burger

Chef salad

Grilled chicken Caesar club sandwich

Bulls-eye BBQ deluxe burger

Santa Fe fire-grilled chicken baguette

Smoky BBQ chicken baguette

Kentucky Fried Chicken
Honey BBQ chicken sandwich

Oven roasted strips meal

Tender roast chicken breast – no skin

BBQ baked beans and corn on the cob

Garden rice and green beans

Mashed potatoes

McDonald's
Apple bran muffin

Egg McMuffin

Hamburger or cheeseburger

Chicken McGrill

McDonald's (cont.)
Grilled chicken Caesar salad

Chef salad

Chicken fajita

Chunky chicken salad

Fruit 'n walnut salad

McLean deluxe

McVeggie burger

Fruit 'n yogurt parfait

Subway
Ham and egg breakfast sandwich

Ham, roast beef, turkey, or roasted chicken breast sandwich

Red wine vinaigrette sub sandwich

Veggie delight sandwich

Sweet onion chicken teriyaki sandwich

Steak and chicken wrap

Salads with ham, turkey, or roasted chicken breast

Chicken noodle, vegetable beef, or minestrone soup

Taco Bell
Chicken, beef, or steak taco or soft taco

Bean burrito

Chicken, beef, or steak burrito supreme, Fresco style

Chicken, beef, or steak fiesta burrito, Fresco style

Chicken, beef, or steak Enchirito, Fresco style

Chicken, beef, or steak Gordita Baja, Fresco style

Rice and refried beans

Tip #73: Road Fuel

When you're traveling on the road, eating healthy can be a challenge. Stopping at fast food restaurants may be the fastest, easiest bet when you're in a hurry, and you can make healthy choices at most of these stops (see Tips #71 and #72). You can also plan ahead so you've got quick snacks on hand to eat when you need energy and no food can be found.

Whenever possible, pack a bag of high-energy snacks the night before you leave. Take your own individual cooler. Include granola bars, sports bars, cereal bars, dried fruit, fresh fruit, juice boxes, crackers, and cereal. These snacks might be just the thing to tide you over when you need quick energy before competition, between games or matches, or if you have to get an early start to the day. See Tip #76 for ideas of foods to pack in your cooler.

During a break in the action, make a grocery store run for apples, bananas, oranges, grapes, yogurt, cheese sticks, baby carrots, and juices. Most grocery stores also have

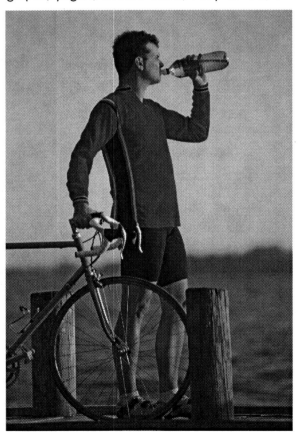

deli sections where you can find low-fat sandwiches that are already prepared. Choose lean meats like turkey, chicken, or lean roast beef. Don't forget one of the most important things of all—drink plenty of juice, water, and sports drinks during the day to stay well-hydrated. A little bit of planning ahead of time can be the difference between making an early exit from a tournament or winning in the finals!

Tip #74: Traveling Tips for a Healthy Trip

When traveling, you need to pay special attention to the liquids you drink and the foods you eat, especially when traveling outside of the country. The following tips will help you decrease your chances of falling prey to an upset digestive tract:

- Bring or buy bottled water whenever possible.
- Bring or buy sports drinks you are used to drinking during training.
- Plan to eat at restaurants that are recommended to you or known to be safe.
- Beware of buffets—the food may have been sitting on the buffet tables for longer than recommended, and that could lead to food poisoning. If you do eat at a buffet, choose foods that are kept at the coldest or hottest temperatures. For instance, if choosing a cold salad, spoon out the salad from the area nearest the ice. When choosing a hot item, look for the "steamiest" dish.
- If competing in a foreign country, consider packing your favorite pre-game foods, such as energy bars or drinks you frequently use.
- Keep the timing of meals and snacks as normal as possible so you don't disrupt your training and eating schedule. Avoid eating too late, or going too long without eating, as it may trigger an upset stomach.
- Always ask for items well-cooked. Eating raw foods or undercooked foods puts you at a greater risk of contracting food poisoning.
- If purchasing food from an area food market once you're at your destination, check the dates on foods to ensure you're not buying foods that are past their expiration dates.
- If flying to your destination, always drink plenty of water before, during, and after the flight to stay hydrated. You lose more fluid at high altitudes, so it's important to plan ahead to keep your body working at its best.

Tip #75: Tournament Fueling

Athletes who play in tournaments that last all day or all weekend long can use the following game plan to get ready for the tournament and keep their energy up all day:

The Night Before the Tournament

Start out with a high-energy meal the night before the tournament. You'll have more fuel stored in your muscles for the next day's performance. Some good ideas:

- Spaghetti with meat sauce, garlic bread, steamed broccoli, strawberries, and low-fat milk
- Thick-crust pizza with ham and veggies with a side salad and low-fat milk or lemonade
- Turkey and cheese sandwich on whole wheat bread, corn, fresh fruit salad, low-fat milk, and oatmeal cookies
- Grilled chicken breast, mashed potatoes, green beans, applesauce, and low-fat milk
- Chicken, vegetable, and rice stir-fry, wonton soup, orange slices, and 100% juice

The Day of the Tournament

Get up early on the day of the tournament and eat a good breakfast. Eat at least two to three hours before you compete. Try the following:

- Pancakes, lean ham slices, a banana, orange juice, and water
- Oatmeal with low-fat milk and raisins, toast with jam, grape juice, and water
- Bagel with peanut butter, melon, apple juice, and water
- Scrambled eggs, English muffins, fruit salad, and orange juice

During the Tournament

- Keep water and sports drinks handy. Drink at least 6-12 ounces every 15-20 minutes during play. For short breaks (15-45 minutes), go for liquids like juices, sports drinks, and extra water.
- For one- to two-hour breaks between matches, try cereal bars, low-fat granola bars, dry cereal, pretzels, graham crackers, fig bars, pudding cups, cheese sticks, bananas, grapes, oranges, yogurt, and juices.
- For longer breaks (two hours or more), try sports bars, lean turkey, chicken, or ham sandwiches, peanut butter and jelly sandwiches, apples, bananas, grapes, oranges, granola bars, yogurt, and juices. The longer you have between competitions, the more you can eat and the more time you have to digest the food without slowing you down (see Tip #64).

Tip #76: Filling the Cooler

Athletes often perform at their best when they think ahead and have a variety of foods available, no matter where or when the competition takes place. Don't rely on the snack bars, concession stands, or fast-food stops to meet all of your nutritional requirements. Team members or parents can take turns filling and bringing two coolers of nutritious snacks for day-long tourneys or competitions to ensure athletes stay well-hydrated and full of energy. Fill one cooler with ice and cold foods, and the other with snack foods that don't need to stay on ice.

Fill up the cold cooler with:

- Bottled water
- Sports drinks
- Liquid meals
- 100% juices
- Yogurt cups and squeeze tubes
- Pudding cups
- Mozzarella cheese sticks
- Cheese cubes
- Lean ham, turkey, or roast beef sandwiches
- Peanut butter sandwiches
- Oranges, apples, grapes, peaches, cherries, and pears
- Fresh, cleaned vegetables such as carrots, celery, peppers, and cauliflower

Fill up the dry-foods cooler with:

- Energy bars
- Cereal bars
- Granola bars
- Fig cookies
- Graham crackers
- Rice cakes
- Soy nuts
- Pretzels
- Animal crackers
- Oatmeal cookies
- GORP (whole grain cereal mixed with nuts and dried fruit)
- Raisins and 100% fruit leather
- Dried apples, pineapple, apricots, and bananas

Tip #77: Time-Saving Kitchen Tips

One reason we may forego eating a sound sports diet to fuel our bodies is because we think we don't have enough time to prepare healthy meals. Fortunately, eating well doesn't need to take a lot of time and energy. But you do want to be smart when you grocery shop, organize your kitchen, and plan meals and snacks. A few extra minutes ahead of time makes it easy to eat well without a lot of hassle.

You should keep the following staples in the kitchen to help you have options for quick meals:

In the refrigerator:
- Orange juice with calcium
- Skim or 1% milk or flavored milk
- Low-fat shredded cheese
- Mozzarella cheese sticks
- Low-fat soy milk and soy cheese
- Boiled eggs
- Single-serving yogurts
- Pre-cut fresh vegetables (broccoli, cauliflower, peppers)
- Pre-made salad mix (with dark lettuce)
- Pre-made cole slaw and broccoli slaw
- Baby carrots
- Fresh fruit like grapes, oranges, grapefruit, apples, and strawberries
- Low-fat salad dressing
- Lean deli meat such as turkey, ham, and roast beef
- Natural peanut butter

In the freezer:
- 100% fruit juices
- Bagged frozen fruit for smoothies (peaches, berries, banana pieces)
- Frozen vegetables
- Lean meat in single-size portions (chicken breasts, meat patties, pork loins)
- Veggie burgers
- Extra bagels, whole grain bread, and English muffins
- Whole grain waffles and pancakes
- Low-fat frozen meals and entrées (see Tip #78)
- Low-fat frozen bean or bean-and-beef burritos
- Ice milk or frozen yogurt

In the pantry:

- Whole grain cold cereals
- Oatmeal
- Whole grain crackers
- Low-fat microwave popcorn
- Cereal bars and granola bars
- Dried fruit like raisins, prunes, apples, and apricots
- Single-serving canned fruit and vegetable juices
- Canned fruit and vegetables
- Nuts, seeds, and soy nuts
- Canned beans
- Packaged bean and rice mixes
- Canned and dried low-fat soups
- Whole grain rice
- Pasta and pasta sauce
- White potatoes and sweet potatoes
- Boxed instant potatoes
- Boxed meals
- Sports drinks, sports bars, and energy drinks

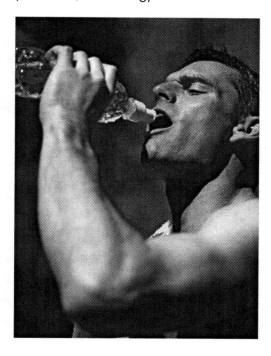

Tip #78: Choosing Frozen Meals and Entrées

The frozen food aisle offers many excellent choices for quick, healthy meals that you can keep on hand to save time and energy when coming home from a hard workout. Use the frozen meal as the base of your lunch or dinner, and add extra items to it to round it out. For instance, if you have a frozen meal consisting of chicken and rice, top it off with steamed fresh broccoli, whole grain bread, and a low-fat vanilla yogurt mixed with fresh strawberries. You've got a meal ready to go in 5-10 minutes.

Look for frozen meals or entrees with 30% or fewer of the calories from fat and at least 10-15 grams of protein. Depending on your daily energy requirements, you may need to heat up two meals to supply enough food. An example of a low-fat meal that also provides a good protein source is Healthy Choice" Lemon Pepper Fish (with rice medley, mixed vegetables, and apple cherry dessert):

> Calories: 320
> Total fat: 7 grams (20% fat)
> Carbohydrate: 50 grams
> Protein: 14 grams

11 recommended frozen meals or entrées:

- Amy's® Santa Fe Enchilada Bowl
- Budget Gourmet® Beef Pepper Steak with Rice
- Chef's Choice® Shrimp Linguine
- Healthy Choice® Lemon Pepper Fish
- Michelina's® Low-fat Black Bean Chili
- Mrs. Paul's® Shrimp Stir Fry Bowl
- Stouffer's Lean Cuisine® Honey Roasted Pork
- Ethnic Gourmet® Pad Thai with Tofu
- Uncle Ben's® Parmesan Shrimp Penne Pasta Bowl
- Weight Watchers Smart Ones® Fiesta Chicken
- Seapoint Farms® Edamame Rice Bowl

Tip #79: Best Bets at Convenience Stops

If your only option for finding healthy snacks to energize your body for a game or refuel after competition is a vending machine, a convenience store, or a "super" gas station, you can still come up with some items that can keep you going strong. You might have to peer behind the rows of doughnuts, candy bars, and sodas, but some healthy options do exist. Keep in mind that you want to meet your total energy needs while finding good carbohydrate and protein sources as well. In addition, you want to maximize the nutrients in foods and drinks you consume, so think about getting a variety of foods from all of the food groups.

Try the following sample snacks to energize you on from a convenience store stop:

- Pre-made turkey, chicken, roast beef, or ham sandwiches
- Low-fat bean burritos
- Low-fat frozen pocket sandwiches
- Microwave popcorn
- Graham crackers
- Animal crackers
- Cheese/peanut butter and cracker combos
- Cereal bars
- Granola bars
- Trail mix
- Pretzels
- Dried fruit
- Fresh fruit
- Yogurt
- Mozzarella cheese sticks
- Soy nuts
- Nuts and seeds (e.g., sunflower seeds or peanuts)
- 100% fruit juices
- Bottled waters
- Low-fat or skim milk or soy milk
- Sports drinks, energy drinks, and sports bars

Tip #80: Checking Out Food Labels

When you're focused on eating to fuel your sports body, understanding food labels is important. The following chart explains some of the common label claims you'll find on foods in your supermarket. Explanations are "per serving."

Label Nutrient Content Claims	Explanation (per serving)
Calorie-free	Under 5 calories
Low calorie	40 calories or less
Reduced or lower	At least 25% less of a nutrient or calories than the regular product
Light or lite	1/3 fewer calories, 50% less sodium, or 50% less fat
Sugar free	Less than 0.5 grams of sugar
Fat-free	Less than 0.5 grams of fat
Trans fat-free	Less than 0.5 grams of trans fat
Low fat	3 grams of fat or less
Cholesterol-free	Under 2 milligrams of cholesterol with no more than 2 grams of saturated fat
Low-cholesterol	20 milligrams or less of cholesterol and 2 grams or less of saturated fat
Lean	Meats, poultry, and fish with less than 10 grams of fat, less than 4.5 grams of saturated fat, and less than 95 milligrams of cholesterol per 3 1/2 ounce cooked serving
Extra lean	Meat, poultry, and fish with under 5 grams of total fat, 2 grams of saturated fat, and 95 milligrams of cholesterol per 3 1/2 ounce cooked serving
Low sodium	No more than 140 milligrams per serving
Very low sodium	No more than 35 milligrams per serving
Good source of vitamins or minerals	Provides 10 to 19 percent or more of Daily Value of that vitamin or mineral per serving
High in	Provides 20 percent or more of the Daily Value of the specified nutrient per serving
High fiber	5 or more grams of fiber per serving
More	A serving of food contains a nutrient that is at least 10 percent of the Daily Value more than the reference food.
Healthy	Low in fat and saturated fat with limited sodium and cholesterol. Most healthy foods must provide at least 10 percent of the Daily Value of vitamin A, vitamin C, iron, protein, calcium, or fiber.
Organic	Produced without using most conventional pesticides; fertilizers made with synthetic ingredients or sewage sludge; bioengineering; or ionizing radiation. USDA's organic seal means the product is at least 95% organic.

11

Special Considerations

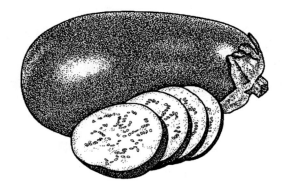

"Athletes who may be more susceptible to muscle cramping often have a low dietary salt intake, lose a lot of electrolytes in their sweat, and perspire at a high rate."

Tip #81: The Vegetarian Athlete

Athletes can meet their nutritional needs while choosing a vegetarian diet. The more restrictive your vegetarian plan is, the more attention you need to pay to your diet to ensure you are getting all of the nutrients you need. You may decide on a vegetarian diet based on your concerns for health, the environment, animal rights, or simply to find a plan that is plant-based. Many studies have found that vegetarians also tend to pay more attention to other areas of their health, such as exercise, so it may be an entire lifestyle approach for you. Whatever your reasons for being or considering becoming a vegetarian, choosing a well-balanced nutrition plan is essential. By doing so, you will reap the health benefits of a vegetarian diet, such as a decreased risk of heart disease and certain cancers, while boosting your sports performance.

Some vegetarians prefer to avoid all animal products, while others limit one or more types of animal foods. Some examples include:

- Semi-vegetarians: avoid red meats but eat some fish, eggs, chicken, turkey, and dairy foods
- Pesco-vegetarians: eat fish, milk products, and eggs
- Lacto-ovo vegetarians: eat milk products and eggs
- Ovo-vegetarians: eat eggs
- Vegans: eat no animal foods at all

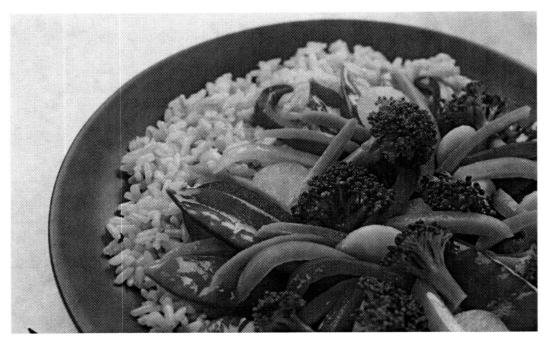

Tip #82: Nutrients for Vegetarians

If you choose vegetarianism, you need to keep an eye out for some important nutrients, including protein, calcium, and iron.

Protein

As an athlete, your protein needs are higher than non-athletes. You need between 0.5 and 0.8 grams of protein daily per pound of body weight (see Tip #21). That's about 45-72 grams for a 90-pound athlete, 60-96 grams for a 120-pound athlete, 75-120 grams for a 150-pound athlete, or 90-144 grams for a 180-pound athlete.

Protein is made from building blocks called amino acids. Some foods have all of the essential amino acids: meat, poultry, eggs, fish, milk, cheese, and yogurt. Other foods are considered very high-quality protein, such as soy foods like tofu, soy milk, or soy nuts. Additional good sources of protein are nuts, peanut butter, seeds like sunflower seeds, and beans, like chili beans or refried beans in burritos. Grains and vegetables also provide smaller amounts of protein in the diet. Sports bars and some energy drinks can also be excellent protein sources. See Tip #23 for more non-animal protein sources.

The key is to get a variety of different foods in your diet each day so you can meet all of these amino acid requirements even if you limit or don't eat any animal products. That way, even if some foods you eat are missing an amino acid, you'll get it in other foods you eat that day.

Calcium

Calcium is one of the key minerals for an athlete. It helps build and maintain strong bones. Some of the best natural sources of calcium are milk and milk products like cheese, yogurt, and milkshakes. Athletes who choose to use milk products generally don't have a problem getting enough calcium if they consume 3-4 servings a day. If milk products are eliminated from the diet, the best places to find calcium are juices, cereals, breads, grain products, waffles fortified with calcium, or calcium-fortified soy products like fortified soy milk, soy cheese, and tofu. Other good sources are oranges, broccoli, turnip and mustard greens, pinto beans, and dried figs. See Tip #35 for more high-calcium ideas.

Iron

Iron is extremely important for an athlete. This mineral is used to form hemoglobin and myoglobin, compounds in the body that carry oxygen in the blood and muscle. If you don't get enough iron in your diet, you may not be able to get adequate oxygen to your muscles during exercise, leading to low energy. The iron found in animal foods (heme iron), particularly red meat, is absorbed best by the body. So, if you don't eat meat, you have to be sure to eat other foods that are good sources of iron, such as eggs, beans, pumpkin seeds, spinach, soy nuts, fortified tofu, raisins, or breads and cereals fortified with 100% iron. Include a food high in Vitamin C, like an orange, kiwi, or tomato juice, to enhance iron absorption. See Tip #37 for more high-iron sources.

Tip #83: Top Vegetarian Foods*

Top 5 Vegetarian Foods for Protein:

Veggie burgers
Tempeh
Soy milk
Peanut butter
Beans (legumes)

Top 5 Vegetarian Foods for Calcium:

Calcium-fortified orange juice
Calcium-fortified cereal
Soy milk with calcium
Tofu with calcium
Calcium-fortified breads

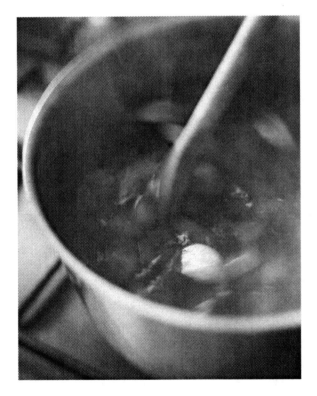

Top 5 Vegetarian Foods for Iron:

Iron-fortified cereals
Iron-fortified breads
Vegetarian chili
Baked beans
Broccoli

As recommended by the author

Tip #84: Hands-On Vegetarian

Vegetarian (vegan) sports nutritionist and endurance athlete Heather Hedrick, MS, RD, shares her recommendations for incorporating a vegetarian diet into an athletic lifestyle.

Question: When you first became vegetarian, did you have to pay special attention to getting in enough specific foods or nutrients?

Answer: The more I learned about a vegetarian diet, the more improvements I made in my diet. Eventually, I created a more balanced diet to obtain all the nutrients I need. As an athlete, I do pay attention to getting enough protein, calcium, iron, and zinc, but with a balanced diet throughout the day, it is easy to meet my needs.

Question: What are some nutrition roadblocks you've faced as a vegetarian?

Answer: Eating out—It can be hard to find vegan foods when eating out. I have found a couple favorite places with vegetarian/vegan foods, and I frequent those restaurants. Otherwise, I prefer to prepare food at home.

Traveling—Traveling has been very challenging, but not impossible. Since I race all over the country and overseas, I have had the opportunity to be creative in making sure that I am still meeting my nutritional needs, but also eating foods I'm comfortable with right before competitions. I bring a lot of food with me. That way I don't need to worry about what I can find at my destination.

Eating at other people's homes—I don't like to inconvenience others by asking them to prepare special food for me, but I also do not want to be rude by refusing to eat what my friends or family have prepared. I have found that a combination of letting them know my restrictions and being flexible works best. I can usually find vegetables, fruits, or bread/grains to eat while skipping the meat and dairy foods within the meal.

Question: What nutrients do you think young vegetarian athletes need to pay special attention to?

Answer: The biggest thing is remembering that if a food is eliminated from the diet, a replacement must be found. If meat is eliminated, then foods like soy products, beans, lentils, or nuts must be placed in the diet. If milk/dairy is eliminated, then soy milk or soy yogurt can be consumed in its place.

Question: Do you have any tips for coaches/athletic trainers/nutritionists working with athletes who are vegetarian?

Answer: Be sensitive to their special needs and desires, especially when traveling or dining together. Find a way for them to get the foods they need, or make arrangements for them to bring their own food in coolers.

Question: Any last suggestions?

Answer: Focus on balance and variety. Have balance at every meal. Eating enough food may not be a problem for most athletes, but they need to make sure it is quality food. Focus on whole foods. So many sports nutrition products, such as bars, powders, and drinks, are on the market. Use them in moderation and make sure to get plenty of fruits, veggies, whole grains, and meat/dairy alternative products so you have a balanced diet.

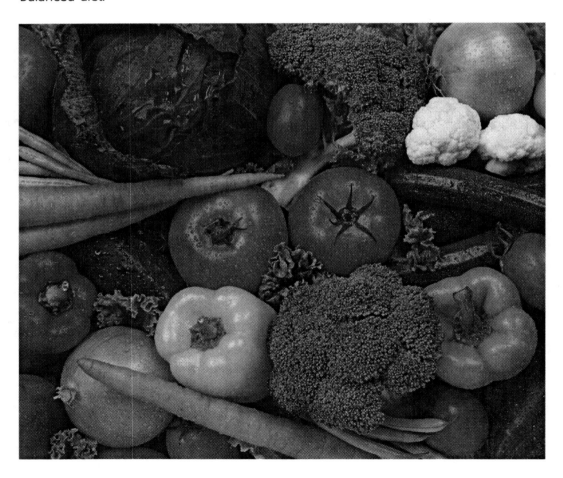

Tip #85: Endurance Nutrition

You're training hard for that next endurance competition. As you move up the ladder with the time and distance you train, your nutrition plan becomes even more important. If you are a runner, you may be able to reach your goals by adding primarily extra fluids with your 5Ks or shorter runs. But once you move into the 10Ks, half-marathons, and marathons, how you fuel your body becomes more and more crucial to your success (and recovery). As you train longer, your body uses more energy, particularly carbohydrate calories. While a strength athlete can often get by on 2-3 grams of carbohydrate per pound of body weight, endurance runners need at least 3-4 grams of carbohydrate per pound per day (see Tip #12). For a 160-pound runner at an ideal body weight range, that's 480-640 grams per day (or 1920-2560 carbohydrate calories) in heavy training. To get your body ready to go for your next endurance race, keep the following tips in mind:

- Consistently eat a high-carbohydrate diet. If your muscles are trained to store carbohydrate energy, you'll have more fuel available at the end of the race. High-carbohydrate foods include breads and cereals, rice, pasta, fruits and fruit juice, vegetables (especially potatoes and corn), peas and beans, yogurt, frozen yogurt, and sweets. Formulated drinks, bars, and gels are also high in carbohydrates. Make these foods the base of your diet while including a high-protein food with your meals. An example of a high-carbohydrate meal with adequate protein is grilled chicken breast, rice, steamed broccoli, whole grain roll, and skim milk with strawberries over frozen yogurt for dessert.

- When you plan your workouts, keep nutrition in mind. Opt for a high-carbohydrate meal two to three hours before your workout, and make sure you are well-hydrated going into the run. Be sure to hydrate before, during, and after your training sessions.

- During your runs, experiment with different sports drinks, gels, and solids to see what works best for you. Most athletes tolerate a lower carbohydrate drink best (14-16 grams of carbohydrate per 8 ounces), but some runners have no intestinal problems taking in 20 grams of carbohydrate per 8 ounces. Try different gels and solids to see what you can handle and what tastes best to you. Remember: when using gels, sports bars, or solids, you must take in extra water. Whether you find sports drinks, gels, solids, or a combination works best for you, the carbohydrate intake goal is 30-60 grams per hour of running. For example, using Gatorade®, that's drinking at least 16-32 ounces per hour.

- Post-workout or post-race fuel: Take in at least 50 grams of carbohydrate within 15-30 minutes (i.e., 3-4 cups of a sports drink or 2 cups lemonade). Adding a small amount of protein (10-15 grams) may also enhance tissue repair (see Tip #67). Next, continue to eat and refuel your muscles within the next few hours to help replenish muscle carbohydrate (glycogen) faster. For example, within two hours after the workout or race, eat a high-carbohydrate meal like a submarine sandwich, fruit, and pretzels. And don't forget to keep the fluids coming after a workout or race. Keep drinking until you're consistently producing a good amount of clear urine.

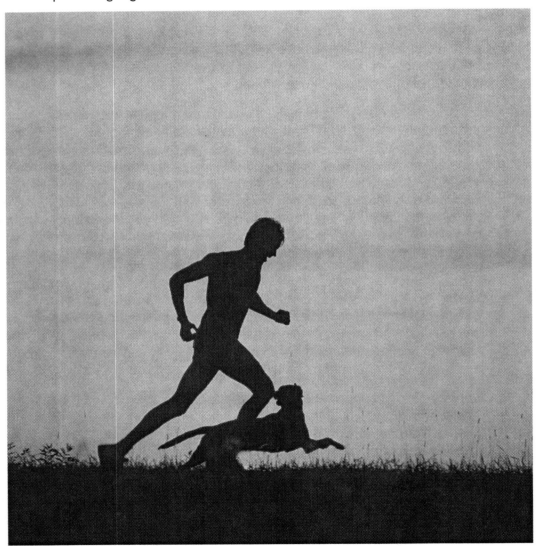

Tip #86: High-Altitude Nutrition

If you're planning to head up to the mountains for your next excursion, a proper sports nutrition plan could be crucial to your success. Because less oxygen is available at high altitudes (especially with rapid ascents to altitudes over 8,000 feet or 2,400 meters), some hikers experience acute mountain sickness (AMS). The symptoms of AMS (headache, fatigue, nausea, and dizziness) can often lead to a decrease in appetite. Think ahead and keep the following tips in mind before you take off on your next high-altitude adventure.

- Enlist your entire team of hikers to develop a nutrition plan before leaving. You'll want to encourage each other to eat enough and get plenty of fluids. Nutrition is a serious part of the success of the venture. Work with a sports nutritionist to develop food plans and keep a log when you hike to know you are on target.

- Stay hydrated. You may need to drink as much as 12 to 20 cups of fluid per day or more to stay in fluid balance. Body fluids are lost more readily at high altitudes. Use your urine as a monitor to be sure you are hydrating appropriately. You should be producing plenty of urine with a pale yellow color.

- Eat enough calories with a good balance of carbohydrates, protein, and fat. Because altitude increases the body's need for energy, many hikers need to eat between 4,000 and 6,000 calories per day to maintain weight when on the mountain. If you don't eat enough, your performance can quickly be compromised, making it more difficult to reach your goals.

Top Foods for the Trek

Powdered sport drink mixes	Freeze dried meals and packaged foods
Powdered high-calorie recovery drink mixes	Instant mashed potatoes, rice, and pasta mixes
Instant lemonade and juice drink mixes	Powdered milk and instant breakfast drinks
Instant cocoa and pudding mixes	
Dried fruit and fruit leather	Instant soup and hot cereal mixes
Powdered eggs	Trail mix, nuts, and hard candy
Peanut butter (may freeze at high altitude)	Fig and fruit bars
	Granola bars and sports bars

Tip #87: Preventing Muscle Cramps

Sweat losses are mostly water, but contain many minerals as well. Although individual athletes lose different concentrations of minerals in sweat, most athletes lose more sodium and chloride than other minerals. Potassium, calcium, and magnesium may also be lost in sweat. Athletes who are acclimated to the heat tend to lose less sodium than those who are not used to exercising in hot weather.

Heat cramps often occur with heavy, repeated sweating. More often than not, they arise at the end of a long day of competition (such as the last soccer match of the day or the finals of a tennis tournament). Athletes who may be more susceptible to muscle cramping often have a low dietary salt intake, lose high amounts of electrolytes in their sweat and perspire at a high rate.

When replenishing your body with fluids and food during or after competition, it's important to take in enough electrolytes. If you sweat a lot, work out in extreme heat, or are prone to muscle cramps, stay well-hydrated and consider adding more electrolytes to your diet using the following methods:

- Salt your food, especially after workouts. Each teaspoon of salt has over 2,300 milligrams of sodium. You'll get almost 600 milligrams for every 1/4 teaspoon you use.

- Choose salty foods or drinks when you eat after workouts. Include foods like salted pretzels, tomato juice, canned soups, canned vegetables, soy sauce, cheese, or frozen items (i.e., frozen dinners and frozen pizza).

- Include foods high in potassium, such as potatoes, tomato juice, orange juice, bananas, canned beans, raisins, trail mix, spinach, pork chops, and milk.

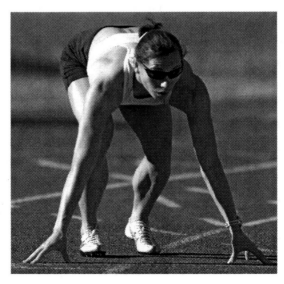

Tip #88: Maximizing Your Nutrient Intake

As an athlete, all of the extra things you do add up and combine to make a positive difference in your sports performance and health. The first step is learning about nutrition and how it can affect your performance and health. Next, you need to make an effort to purchase, prepare, and eat a variety of nutritious foods. How you do that can make an impact on the quality of your diet. The following quick tips can help you maximize your intake:

- Choose fruits and vegetables in season in your area. They are often fresher and of higher nutritional quality than out-of-season items.

- Shop at local farmers markets to take advantage of fresh produce.

- Choose smaller, brightly colored produce as opposed to larger produce with a washed-out color. Check produce to avoid fruits and vegetables that are blemished.

- Go for organic foods when possible if your budget and shopping opportunities allow for it.

- Go for whole grains as much as possible. Choose whole wheat pasta, brown rice, and whole grain breads, rolls, and bagels.

- Look for a high fiber content on grains. These items are most likely to be made from whole grains.

- Use fresh herbs to enhance the flavor of foods and lend extra vitamins, minerals, and natural plant chemicals to your diet.

- Check expiration dates on items to be sure you are buying fresh foods. Get in the habit of choosing items from the back of the row, as these are generally the most recent ones stocked.

- Plan your grocery shopping trips into your weekly schedule. The more often you shop, the better able you are to have a variety of fresh, high-quality food choices available.

Tip #89: Phytochemicals and Functional Foods

Phytochemicals are plant chemicals (phyto means plant) that may offer a particular nutritional benefit. Functional foods are foods that pack an extra nutritional punch. These foods may have nutritional benefits that go beyond basic nutrition, or beyond what we generally think of as typical vitamins and minerals. The key with functional foods is that what you *do* eat may benefit you more than what you *don't* eat. In other words, the message is a positive one. Instead of thinking of cutting foods out of your diet to improve your health, you actually focus on eating more of these particular foods, which are often loaded with phytochemicals or zoochemicals (animal sources of healthy compounds).

Although all foods are functional in one way or another, consider boosting your intake of foods that have been found to contain the "bonus" nutrients listed in the following chart. Many of these foods are plant-based, giving you yet another good reason to load up your diet with plant foods like fruits, vegetables, and whole grains. The potential benefits from eating these foods are vast.

Class of Phytochemicals or Zoochemicals and Examples	Examples of Food Sources	Potential Benefits to Eating these Functional Foods
Carotenoids Beta-carotene, lutein, lycopene, zeaxanthin	Carrots, leafy green vegetables, tomatoes, tomato paste, citrus fruits	May decrease damage to the body's cells; helps maintain healthy vision (see Tip #90)
Flavonoids Anthocyanadins, catechins, flavones, sulphoraphane	Fruits, vegetables, tea	May decrease damage to the body's cells; may reduce the risk of certain cancers; may decrease risk of cardiovascular disease
Fatty Acids Omega-3 fatty acids, conjugated linoleic acid (CLA)	Tuna, salmon, herring, flax; cheese, meat products (CLA)	May reduce the risk of cardiovascular disease; may improve body composition; may decrease the risk of certain cancers
Prebiotics / Probiotics Fructo-oligosaccharides (FOS); lactobacillus	Yogurt, kefir, onion powder, shallots, Jerusalem artichokes	May improve gastrointestinal health
Sulfides Diallyl sulfide	Onions, garlic, scallions, leeks	May lower LDL cholesterol; may help maintain immune health
Tannins Proanthocyanidins	Cranberries, blueberries, chocolate	May enhance urinary tract health; may reduce the risk of cardiovascular disease
Soy Protein	Soybeans, soy milk, tofu, tempeh	May reduce the risk of heart disease

For a more detailed look at functional foods, visit the International Food Information Council Foundation (www.ific.org) website.

Tip #90: Eating for Healthy Eyes

As an athlete, having keen eyesight is an added advantage in most sports. So eating foods that may promote healthy eyes is a positive step you can take to be on top of your game. In the last few years, many research studies have pointed to important foods and nutrients that play a role in maintaining healthy eyes, especially as we age. Take a close look at these tips for keeping your eyes on target.

Choose foods high in lutein and zeaxanthin. Eating foods high in these two food components is linked to preventing the eye disease macular degeneration, the leading cause of blindness as we age. Add more lutein and zeaxanthin to your diet by consuming more dark, leafy green vegetables like spinach, broccoli, collard greens, and kale. Add these dark greens to salads, or stir-fry them with onions and carrots and eat with high-fiber brown rice.

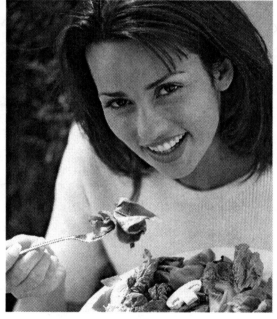

Eat more pasta sauce and other foods high in lycopene. Lycopene is a natural food chemical found in high amounts in tomato products like tomato sauce, tomato paste, tomato juice, salsa, and chili sauce. It's also present in smaller amounts in other foods like watermelon and pink grapefruit. Studies have linked lycopene intake with a decreased risk of developing cataracts, an eye problem that affects as many as half of all people over the age of 65.

Eat more antioxidants, especially Vitamin C. Consuming a diet high in antioxidants is a key to keeping your eyes healthy. Aim for a minimum of six servings of fruits and vegetables a day. Eat more citrus fruits and juices, peppers, strawberries, kiwi fruit, and potatoes for starters. See Tip #35 for more Vitamin C-rich foods.

Tip: To find lists of foods high in lutein, zeaxanthin, and lycopene, check out the United States Department of Agriculture Nutrient Database for carotenoids website at http://www.nal.usda.gov/fnic/foodcomp/Data/car98/car98.html. Then click on "data table."

Tip #91: Lactose Intolerance

Lactose is a natural sugar (ose means sugar) found in milk and milk products. People with lactose intolerance make too little lactase (the enzyme that digests lactose) to properly break down the milk sugar. When lactose is not fully digested, it is fermented in the small intestine and can cause bloating, cramping, abdominal pain, gas, nausea, and diarrhea.

Some people can handle small amounts of lactose at a time (e.g., 1/2 cup of milk) without problems, while others find avoiding milk products altogether is most beneficial. As an athlete, you don't want lactose intolerance to be hindering your performance. If you're concerned about lactose intolerance, keep an eye on the foods you eat that contain lactose and find out how much your body can tolerate.

On the food label, check for the following ingredients: milk, dry milk, dry milk solids, milk chocolate, lactose, buttermilk, malted milk, sour cream, cheese, whey, and margarine. Packaged foods like pancake mixes, muffin mixes, salad dressings, cream soup mixes, instant noodle or potato mixes, and frozen pizza also contain lactose.

Don't just drop all dairy products from your diet if you're lactose intolerant. You may be able to eat small amounts of these foods. In addition, foods like yogurt with active cultures (check the label) have "friendly" bacteria that make it easier to digest. When choosing cheeses, look for aged cheeses (like Swiss, colby, parmesan, and cheddar), as they have much of the lactose removed in processing.

Foods high in lactose	Lactose-free foods
Sweetened condensed milk	Fruits and fruit juices
Evaporated milk	Vegetables (without added sauces)
Milk or buttermilk	Soy milk, soy cheese, tofu, and many other soy products
Nonfat dry milk	
Ice cream or ice milk	Plain meat, fish, and poultry
Yogurt	Many sports bars/drinks without milk
Cheese	Breads, cereals, desserts, packaged products, and snack foods made without milk or milk products
Half-and-half or sour cream	

Tip #92: Ten Tips for Avoiding Food Poisoning

As an athlete, the last thing you need slowing you down is an unfortunate bout with food poisoning. Since more than 100 different types of bacteria can cause foodborne illness, keeping a safe kitchen is a first step in decreasing your risk of food poisoning. Keep the following tips in mind to minimize your risk of food poisoning.

1. Wash your hands with warm, soapy water for at least 20 seconds before preparing food. Wash frequently during food preparation, especially if you're handling raw meats.

2. Keep your kitchen counters and work surfaces clean.

3. Use separate knives and cutting boards for meats, poultry, and seafood, and other foods like veggies and fruits to avoid cross-contamination.

4. Check the expiration dates on foods when you purchase them. Choose items toward the back of the row in the grocery store, as they often post later expiration dates.

5. Wash dishcloths and towels frequently or use disposable ones. Sponges or scouring pads can even be washed in the dishwasher.

6. Put the "doggie bag" in the refrigerator as soon as possible after eating out.

7. Cook meats, poultry, and eggs thoroughly.

8. Keep your refrigerator at 40° F (4°C) and your freezer at 0°F (-18°C). Invest in fridge and freezer thermometers so you can keep an eye on temperatures.

9. Put leftovers in the fridge within two hours of eating.

10. Use leftovers within three to four days or toss.

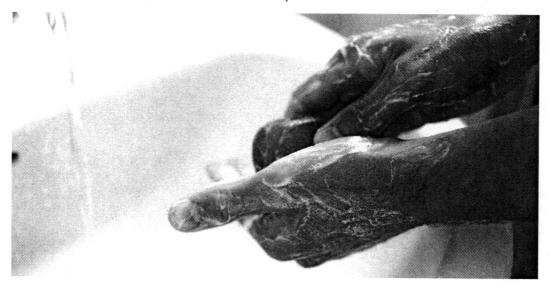

Tip #93: Ideas for Picky Eaters

If you're a picky eater, you may be missing out on important nutrients to help you fuel your fitness. Your body needs enough total energy, protein, carbohydrate, fat, vitamins, minerals, and fluids on a consistent basis to keep going strong. Although you don't need 100% of every nutrient every day, think of your body working on weeks and months at a time. Over the course of a week, you want to achieve a balance of nutrients even if some days you eat better than others.

- If you don't like many vegetables, eat more of the ones you do like. For instance, if you grew up on and still favor the "big three" of Midwestern vegetables (corn, potatoes, and green beans), with an iceberg lettuce salad thrown in for variety now and then, make a point to eat these vegetables more often, and try to make up for lost nutrients by eating other foods, like fruits. Go for more fresh, frozen, or canned fruits and fruit juices for extra Vitamin C and antioxidants. Shoot for a minimum of 5-6 servings of fruits and vegetables a day.

- If you're a picky meat eater, be sure to have at least two good protein sources a day. If you like chicken, buy frozen, skinned chicken breasts or tenderloins, and prepare several at a time so you've got leftovers in the refrigerator. Stock other good protein sources like low-fat cheese, yogurt, canned beans or refried beans, tofu, and eggs. Boil extra eggs so you have them ready to go as a quick protein source.

- Don't be afraid to try new foods. If you're in a rut, try to eat one new food at least once a week. You might find you like foods you never thought you would enjoy. Our tastes change over time, so you might surprise yourself and branch out with your palate if you just give it a try.

- Lastly, don't pass on picky eating habits to your kids, who are easily influenced by what others in the family will and won't eat. Offer a variety of foods to kids and have a positive attitude about food yourself so kids will grow up enjoying and embracing a wide range of foods.

Tip #94: Tips for Coaches and Parents

For young athletes, coaches and parents are in charge of planning and organizing pre-game meals, and making sure athletes are well-nourished before competition. Keep the following tips in mind if you're planning the food for your team members:

- Organize different parents to be in charge of the team coolers for each game or tournament. This way, you can be sure your athletes will have opportunities to eat before, during, and after the games or competitions. Make a list of recommended items (see Tip #76) to include each time so it's easy on the adults making the shopping trip.

- Make a pact to stop for healthy meals whenever possible. Teaching young athletes the importance of fueling their bodies with a variety of high-energy foods is the foundation for developing sound eating habits later in life.

- Be a role model. As a parent or coach, young athletes will model your behavior, be it positive or negative. Many young athletes have started an unhealthy eating practice (such as restrictive dieting) because a coach or parent may have encouraged it or was practicing the unhealthy behavior around the team. Encourage athletes to maintain a well-balanced sports eating plan without restricting certain foods. Bring in a sports nutritionist to talk about specific nutrition recommendations so athletes get sound advice.

- When you arrive at the competition site, scout around to be sure you know where the nearest water fountains are and help your athletes stay well-stocked with water and sports drinks.

- Plan pre-game meals for home and away games and competitions. Schedule pre-game meals at the school or at a parent's or coach's home so all athletes have a chance to eat a good meal regardless of income. These meals are also great team bonding activities.

- Never focus on an athlete's body weight or size, especially in front of other athletes. Even in sports where obtaining a certain body weight is a demand of the sport, treat athletes with respect and confidence to avoid fostering restrictive dieting behaviors or a negative body image.

12

Sample Meal Plans and Resources

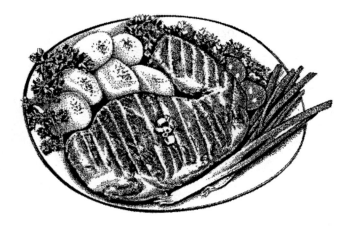

"When seeking advice from sports nutrition professionals, look for those with strong credentials and experience in the field."

Tip #95: Sample 1,800-Calorie Meal Plan

Breakfast

1 cup wheat flakes cereal (e.g., Wheaties)

1 cup skim, 1%, or low-fat soy milk

1 banana

1 slice whole wheat toast

1 tablespoon peanut butter

1 cup 100% orange juice

2 cups water

Lunch

1 turkey sandwich on rye with mozzarella cheese, lettuce, tomato, and light mayonnaise

1 cup baby carrots

1 apple

2 oatmeal cookies

2 cups water

Snack

1/2 cup pretzels

1/4 cup raisins

2 cups water

Dinner

3 ounces lean roast beef

1/2 cup brown rice

1 cup steamed broccoli

1 dinner roll/1 teaspoon margarine

2 cups iced tea

Snack

1 cup low-fat fruit yogurt

2 cups water

Nutrient Breakdown

60% carbohydrate

18% protein

22% fat

Tip #96: Sample 2,200-Calorie Meal Plan

Breakfast
1 cup oatmeal
1 cup skim, 1%, or low-fat soy milk
1 cup low-fat yogurt
1 peach
2 cups water

Lunch
1 tuna sandwich on whole wheat bread
1 pear
1 small package (1 ounce) potato chips
1/2 cup fresh cauliflower
10 animal crackers
2 cups water

Pre-Workout
4 cups sports drink

Post-Workout
1 cup dry cereal with 1 cup skim, 1%, or low-fat soy milk
1 cup grape juice
2 cups water

Dinner
3 ounces grilled chicken breast
1 baked potato with 1 tablespoon light margarine
1 cup steamed mixed vegetables
1 cup spinach salad with 1 tablespoon low-fat dressing
1 cup skim, 1%, or low-fat soy milk
2 cups water

Snack
3 whole grain graham cracker rectangles with 1 tablespoon almond butter
1 cup red grapes
2 cups water

Nutrient Breakdown
63% carbohydrate
14% protein
23% fat

Tip #97: Sample 2,600-Calorie Meal Plan

Breakfast
1 raisin bagel with 2 tablespoons lite cream cheese
1/2 red grapefruit
1 cup whole grain oat cereal (e.g., Cheerios®)
1 cup skim, 1%, or low-fat soy milk
1 cup 100% orange juice
2 cups water

Lunch
2 soft shell chicken tacos
1 serving refried beans
1 serving rice
2 cups iced tea
2 cups water

Pre-workout
1 ounce whole grain crackers
6-ounce nonfat yogurt
2 cups water

Post-workout
1 energy bar
1 orange
2 cups water

Dinner
1 1/2 cups spaghetti with 4 meatballs and sauce
1 cup green beans with 1 teaspoon margarine
1 cup spinach salad with 1 tablespoon regular salad dressing
1 cup skim, 1%, or low-fat soy milk
2 cups water

Snack
3 cups microwave popcorn
1 peach
1 cup apple juice
2 cups water

Nutrient Breakdown
58% carbohydrate
17% protein
25% fat

Tip #98: Sample 3,000-Calorie Meal Plan

Breakfast

2 scrambled eggs

3 slices whole grain toast/ 3 teaspoons margarine

1 cup fresh melon

1 cup skim, 1%, or low-fat soy milk

2 cups water

Lunch

1 cup vegetable bean soup

4 oz. ham and 1 oz. cheese on whole wheat

1 cup pretzel chips

1 1/2 cups fresh fruit salad

2 cups water

Pre-workout

1 whole grain cereal bar

1 banana

2 cups water

Post-workout

1 high-energy drink (e.g., Carnation Instant Breakfast® drink)

2 cups water

Dinner

2 cups tofu and vegetable stir-fry

1 1/2 cups rice

1 cup fresh blueberries with 1 cup low-fat frozen yogurt

2 cups water

Snack

2 cups quick flavored noodles (e.g., ramen)

1 cup skim, 1%, or low-fat soy milk

2 cups water

Nutrient Breakdown

60% carbohydrate

18% protein

22% fat

Tip #99: Sample 3,400-Calorie Meal Plan

Breakfast
4 pancakes with 1 tablespoon margarine
1/4 cup syrup
2 oz. lean ham
1 banana
2 cups grapefruit-orange juice
2 cups water

Lunch
3 oz. grilled black bean burger on a whole grain bun
1 cup fresh pineapple
1 cup cole slaw
2 cups skim, 1%, or low-fat soy milk
2 cups water

Pre-workout
1/2 cup trail mix
6-ounce nonfat yogurt
2 cups water

Post-workout
1 energy bar
1 cup watermelon
2 cups water

Dinner
6 oz. lean grilled pork loin chop
1 cup couscous
1 cup steamed fresh vegetables
1 cup tomato juice
1 whole grain roll with 1 teaspoon margarine
2 cups water

Snack
4 oatmeal raisin cookies
1 cup skim, 1%, or low-fat soy milk

Nutrient Breakdown
60% carbohydrate
18% protein
22% fat

Tip #100: Finding a Sports Nutritionist

If you're seriously looking to make sound, health-based changes in your sports nutrition plan to help you improve performance, you'll want to work with a professional who bases recommendations on accurate, well-researched information. A lot of "quasi-nutritionists" are out there, but don't settle for less than what you deserve. To find a partner who fits you and your goals, look for the following:

- Professionals with a degree in nutrition or dietetics.

- Professionals with R.D. (Registered Dietitian) behind their names. These nutrition professionals have completed a supervised internship program and at least four years of education in nutrition or a related field from a regionally accredited college or university program approved by the American Dietetic Association. In addition, a Registered Dietitian has passed the national accreditation examination. Registered Dietitians are also required to stay current in their education by completing at least 75 hours of continuing education every five years.

- Members of the SCAN (Sports, Cardiovascular, and Wellness Nutritionists) practice group of the American Dietetic Association. Many of these R.D.s specialize in sports and wellness nutrition.

- A member of ACSM (American College of Sports Medicine). Members who are Registered Dietitians generally have expertise and experience in exercise as well as nutrition.

- A professional with an advanced degree in a nutrition, health, or exercise-related field.

- A professional with experience working specifically with athletes.

Note: To find a registered dietitian in your area with experience in sports, log onto the American Dietetic Association's website at www.eatright.org. Enter your zip code at "Find a Nutrition Professional" to search for a specialist near you.

Tip #101: Recommended Health and Nutrition Websites

The following websites are selected recommendations that can be helpful in finding nutrition, health, and fitness information on the web. They are sites that are designed to provide reputable information in an easy-to-use format.

Sports Nutrition
Gatorade Sports Science Institute
www.gssiweb.com

Nutrition on the Move
www.eatnmove.com

Sports and Nutrition: The Winning Connection
www.urbanext.uiuc.edu/hsnut

Nutrition Science & the Olympics
http://btc.montana.edu/olympics/nutrition/

Sports, Fitness, and Nutrition Organizations
American College of Sports Medicine
www.acsm.org

American Dietetic Association
www.eatright.org

IDEA Health and Fitness Association
www.ideafit.com

International Food Information Council Foundation
www.ific.org

National Collegiate Athletic Association
www.ncaa.org

U. S. Government Nutrition Recommendations
Food and Drug Administration
www.fda.gov

Food and Nutrition Information Center
www.nal.usda.gov/fnic

USDA Center for Nutrition Policy and Promotion
www.usda.gov/cnpp

Online Nutrition Analysis Tools

Nutrition Analysis Tools and System
http://nat.crgq.com

United States Department of Agriculture (USDA) Nutrient Data Laboratory
www.nal.usda.gov/fnic/foodcomp/

FatCalories.com
www.fatcalories.com

Dietfacts.com
www.dietfacts.com

Nutrition Website Reviews

Tufts Nutrition Navigator
www.navigator.tufts.edu

Vegetarianism

Vegetarian Resource Group
www.vrg.org

Eating Disorders

National Eating Disorders Association
www.nationaleatingdisorders.org

Something Fishy Website on Eating Disorders
www.somethingfishy.org

Dietary Supplements and Functional Foods

Office of Dietary Supplements
http://dietary-supplements.info.nih.gov/

Natural Medicines Comprehensive Database
www.naturaldatabase.com

Memorial Sloan-Kettering Cancer Center About Herbs, Botanicals, & Other Products
www.mskcc.org/aboutherbs

National Center for Complementary and Alternative Medicine
www.nccam.nih.gov/

ConsumerLab.com
www.consumerlab.com

Supplement Watch
www.supplementwatch.com

International Food Information Council
www.ific.org

General Medical and Health Information

Mayo Clinic
www.mayoclinic.com

InteliHealth
www.intelihealth.com

WebMD
www.webmd.com

Nutrition Action Healthletter
www.cspinet.org/nah/

References

American Academy of Family Physicians. 2002. Sports and women athletes: the female athlete triad. www.familydoctor.org.

American Dietetic Association, Dietitians of Canada, and the American College of Sports Medicine, 2000. Position of the American Dietetic Association, Dietitians of Canada, and the American College of Sports Medicine: Nutrition and Athletic Performance. *Journal of the American Dietetic Association* 100:1543-1546.

Arnett, B., et al., 2001. Speeding recovery from exercise. *Sports Science Exchange Roundtable* 12(4):1-4.

Bergeron, M.F. 2000. Sodium: The forgotten nutrient. *Gatorade Sports Science Exchange* 13(3):1-4.

Brown, R.C. and Cox, C.M. 1998. Effects of high-fat versus high-carbohydrate diets on plasma lipids and lipoproteins in endurance athletes. *Medicine & Science in Sports & Exercise* 30(12):1677-1683.

Burke et al., 2003. Addition of amino acids to sports drinks does not enhance endurance performance. *Medicine & Science in Sports & Exercise*, 35:S211.

Casa, D. J. et al., 2000. National Athletic Trainers' Association Position Statement: Fluid Replacement for Athletes, *Journal of Athletic Training* 35(2):212-224.

Clarkson, P.M. 1998. Nutritional supplements for weight gain. *Gatorade Sports Science Exchange* 11(1):1-6.

Deutz, R., et al., 2000. Relationship between energy deficits and body composition in elite female gymnasts and runners. *Medicine & Science in Sports & Exercise* 32(3):659-667.

Eating for eye health—new research sharpens the focus. 2002. *Tufts University Health & Nutrition Letter* 19(11):4-5.

Eberle, S. 2000. Endurance sports nutrition. Champaign, IL: Human Kinetics.

Food and Drug Administration. The Food Label, *FDA Backgrounder* May 1999, www.cfsan.fda.gov.

Food and Nutrition Board, National Academies of Science. 2004. Dietary reference intake vitamin and mineral tables. www.nationalacademies.org.

Golden NH. 2000. Osteoporosis prevention: A pediatric challenge, *Archives of Pediatrics* 154(6):542-543.

International Food Information Council Foundation. 2004. Functional Foods, www.ific.org.

Krauss, R. et al. 2000. AHA Dietary Guidelines: Revision 2000: A Statement for Healthcare Professionals From the Nutrition Committee of the American Heart Association. *Circulation* 102:2284-2299.

Kundrat, S. 2004. How safe are ephedra-free supplements? *Gatorade Sports Science News*, www.gssiweb.com.

Kundrat, S. 1999. Bugged about food safety? *IDEA Health and Fitness Source*: 17(8):53-57.

Kundrat, S. 1997. Fighting fat phobia. *IDEA Today* 15(4):59-61.

Kundrat, S. 2000. "High-altitude nutrition," SCAN website, www.nutrifit.org/nutrition_information/high_altitude_nutrition.htm.

Manore, M. and Thompson, J. 2000. Sport nutrition for health and performance. Champaign, IL: Human Kinetics.

Margreaves, M. 1999. Carbohydrate ingestion and exercise: effects on metabolism and performance. *Gatorade Sports Science Exchange* 12(4):1-4.

Overweight Overnight. 1998. *ACE Fitness Matters* 4:4.

Poortmans, J. R. and Dellalieux, O. 2000. Do regular high-protein diets have potential health risks on kidney function in athletes? *International Journal of Sport Nutrition and Exercise Metabolism* 10(1):28-35.

Rawson, E.S. and Clarkson, P.M. 2003. Scientifically debatable: is creatine worth its weight? Gatorade Sports Science Exchange 16(4):1-6.

Rosenbloom, C. (ed) 2000. Sports nutrition: a guide for the professional working with active people. Chicago, IL: The American Dietetic Association.

Sarubin, A. 2003. The health professional's guide to dietary supplements. Chicago, IL: The American Dietetic Association.

Smith, A. D. 1996. The female athlete triad. *The Physician and Sportsmedicine*, 24(7):67-76; 86.

United States Department of Agriculture & The United States Department of Health and Human Services. 2000. Nutrition and Your Health: Dietary Guidelines for Americans, 2000.

Venkatraman, J.T. et al. 2000. Dietary fats and immune status in athletics: clinical applications. *Medicine & Science in Sports & Exercise* 32(7):S389-S395.

Vergauwen, L. et al. 1998. Carbohydrate supplementation improves stroke performance in tennis. *Medicine & Science in Sports and Exercise*, 30(8):1289-1295.

Vitamin C: Foods yes, pills no. 1998. *Consumer Reports on Health*, 10(11):1-4.

Walberg R. J. 1997. Glycemic index and exercise metabolism. *Sports Science Exchange* 10(1):1-7.

Williams, M. H. 1998. The ergogenics edge. Champaign, IL: Human Kinetics.

About the Author

Sports nutritionist Susan Kundrat, MS, RD, LD, is the founder and owner of Nutrition on the Move (www.eatnmove.com) in Urbana, Illinois. She specializes in providing sports and wellness nutrition programs for athletes, coaches, health professionals, and the general public. She was named All-Region in three sports (basketball, volleyball, and softball) at Waldorf College. She received her Bachelor's degree in dietetics from Minnesota State University–Mankato, where she was the point guard for the Lady Mavs basketball team. Her master's degree in nutrition is from Iowa State University in Ames.

Susan is the sports nutrition consultant for the Northwestern University Wildcats and the University of Evansville (IN) Purple Aces. From 1993-1998, Susan was the sports nutritionist at the University of Illinois SportWell Center and continues to serve as a consultant for ILLINI athletes including University of Illinois wrestling. She is a member of the Sports Nutrition Board of the Gatorade Sports Science Institute. In addition, Susan is the nutritionist for Strawberry Fields Natural Foods Store in Urbana. She has worked extensively with the University of Illinois Functional Foods for Health Program and is an adjunct lecturer with the Food Science and Human Nutrition Department. She has a monthly nutrition call-in show on local public radio, while her morning nutrition tips are heard weekly on several central Illinois stations.

Susan has 15 years of experience in sports and wellness nutrition and health promotion and is currently a contributing editor for *IDEA Fitness Journal.* She is featured on two training videos, *Sports Nutrition for Teen Athletes* and *Preventing Eating Disorders in Teen Athletes*, from Healthy Learning. She speaks nationally to athletes, health professionals, and coaches on methods to enhance sports performance with optimum nutrition. She is a Registered Dietitian and member of the American Dietetic Association, the American College of Sports Medicine, the Sports, Cardiovascular, and Wellness Nutritionists (SCAN), Nutrition Entrepreneurs, and Nutrition in Complementary Care. In 2003, she was awarded the SCAN Excellence in Practice Award for Sports Nutrition, and in 1997, she was named "Registered Young Dietitian of the Year" by the Illinois Dietetic Association. She and her family enjoy sports and activities of all kinds including cycling, hiking, camping, tennis, swimming, and cross-country skiing.